Praise for Christine Bailey

"What makes Christine unique is her ability to combine her scientific knowledge of nutrition with delicious, gut-healing recipes suitable for everyone. Each recipe is designed to be mind-blowingly tasty and beautiful, yet packed with health-giving nutrients to support your digestive health and promote health and healing."

Dr Mark Hyman, MD, Director, Cleveland Clinic Center for Functional Medicine, author of *The Blood Sugar Solution*

"Who better than Christine Bailey to guide parents through the minefield that is caring for a child with food allergies? Not only does she have professional knowledge to ensure that your child remains well nourished despite the foods that they have to exclude, but she has three highly allergic children of her own – so knows what life at the coalface of food allergy is all about. And as a bonus she is a great cook and creates super-delicious recipes. A must have book."

Michelle Berriedale-Johnson, Director, FreeFrom Food Awards

"Christine...combines the scientific understanding of how our digestive systems work, and importantly why and how they can go wrong, with the creative insight of a smart chef, to produce a fabulous mix of oh-so-tasty recipes that directly support digestive health."

Antony Haynes, BA(Hons), Dip ION, Registered Nutritional Therapist, Functional Medicine Practitioner

"Adverse or out of the ordinary responses to foods are increasing in frequency, particularly in the West. Christine explains the 'why' as well as the 'what to do about it' with healthy, tasty solutions."

Michael Ash, DO, ND, BSc, RNT Functional Medicine Pioneer

Also by Christine Bailey:

The Brain Boost Diet Plan
The Gut Health Diet Plan
The Big Book of Quick, Easy Family Recipes
Go Lean Vegan
The Functional Nutrition Cookbook
The Supercharged Green Juice & Smoothie Diet
The Supercharged Juice & Smoothie Diet
Nourish: The Cancer Care Cookbook

My Kids Can't Eat That!

HOW TO DEAL WITH ALLERGIES & INTOLERANCES IN CHILDREN

CHRISTINE BAILEY

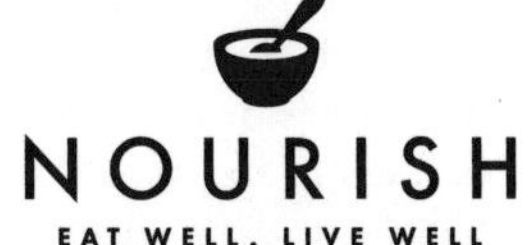

To my three sons: Nathan, Isaac and Simeon, who are my inspiration and motivation in everything I do. Thank you for your encouragement – and for test tasting every recipe in this book numerous times!

This edition published in the UK and USA 2018 by
Nourish, an imprint of Watkins Media Limited
89–93 Shepperton Road
London N1 3DF

enquiries@nourishbooks.com

1 3 5 7 9 10 8 6 4 2

Typeset by seagulls.net

Printed and bound in the UK

A CIP record for this book is available from the British Library

ISBN: 978-1-84899-357-0

www.watkinspublishing.com

Contents

Foreword

My motivation for writing this book is a personal one: this is the book I wish I'd been given when my three boys were young and I first discovered the range of foods that, between them, they aren't able to eat.

For them, and as a coeliac myself, I have learned how to adapt our family life and eating patterns without compromising our health or enjoyment of delicious foods. I feel I am lucky. As a qualified nutritional therapist and a chef, if anyone was going to be able to create homely, appetising and nutritionally balanced allergy-free family recipes, it was me. So many of my clients – and my friends – haven't had the benefit of all that professional training. I want this book to give some of the insight and practical help that I am lucky enough to have just because of what I do.

But, the book is much more than just a great free-from recipe book. I have also trained with the Institute of Functional Medicine, which has meant that I also wanted to include information about why allergies develop. I believe that if you can understand how a food allergy, sensitivity or intolerance works in a child's body, and address the underlying imbalances that are its root cause, you can reduce that child's allergic potential and optimize health for good. While your child may never be able to eat his or her particular allergen foods, with simple dietary and lifestyle changes, it is possible to make dramatic differences to overall health and ensure that he or she grows up strong and full of energy.

All parents want the best for their children. Being diagnosed with a food allergy can feel very daunting not only for a child, but for his or her parents too. That's why I've included plenty of practical advice on living with and taking control of a food allergy – such as how to avoid cross-contamination, cope when travelling, eat safely away from home, and manage parties and family events without anyone feeling like they are missing out.

I also wanted this book to be positive. Instead of focusing on what your child cannot eat, I want you to go away feeling confident enough to explore all the nutritious foods he or she can enjoy. When you cook your family meals from scratch, you'll find that they are tastier, more nutritious and often naturally free-from. I hope that by encouraging you to celebrate the pure joy of eating real food, you and your children are more likely to cook together. Being with you in the kitchen and helping you while you cook, allows children to grow in confidence, and to develop skills and healthy eating habits that will last them a lifetime. One of the greatest joys for me is seeing my own boys making fabulous meals for themselves and others.

I encourage you to read the book from the start, no matter where you are on your child's allergy journey. I hope that every morsel of information is another step to a healthy, nutritionally balanced and utterly delicious future for you and your child.

Introduction

The aim of this book is to guide you through the various types of food reaction that may be affecting your child so that you can not only eliminate culprit foods from your child's diet and substitute in interesting and nutritious ways, but address underlying imbalances in your child's whole body to transform his or her health. This book is divided into three parts.

The first part, "What does it all mean?", breaks down each of the different types of food reactions, their causes and symptoms. I then explain what's happening to your child's immune system, risk factors for each reaction and why the gut plays a crucial role in the development of allergies. This section also includes my route to resolution – how you can identify the underlying imbalances involved in your child's food reactions and symptoms and how to restore balance in order to reduce your child's allergic potential and ongoing symptoms.

The second part, "Getting down to business", looks at how to support your child through diagnosis and living with allergy, both practically and emotionally. It includes guidance on how to talk to your children about their allergies in age-appropriate terms that help them understand what's happening to them and how to manage their allergy themselves (in time, self-management is the greatest gift you can give). There are practical ideas and suggestions about how to cope with food allergies – as a family, and as individuals – in daily life. I'll show you how to avoid cross-contamination, for example, and prepare you for travelling and eating together away from home. I've included plenty of advice about how to work with your child's nursery or school to ensure he or she is safe even when outside your care, and how to ensure your child enjoys birthday parties and other celebrations without feeling excluded or different.

Part two also gives practical and accessible nutritional advice to help you create a nourishing diet for the whole family and ensure your child is not missing out on key nutrients, whatever you have to eliminate. Practically, of course, you also need the skills and information to cook nutritious meals for everyone. By understanding the ingredients to which your child is allergic, and how to avoid or substitute them in your cooking, you'll feel more confident not only in your own ability in the kitchen but, if you cook with your child, learning together as you go, you'll also gain confidence in your child's ability to manage his or her own allergy. Overall, both you and your child will feel more in control of the allergy, and life.

The third part, "Mealtimes in practice", includes a range of meal plans that not only cover gluten-free, dairy-free and egg-free dishes, but those that help lower inflammation, nourish the gut and rebalance the immune system to minimize symptoms. By including nutrient-rich meals that help tackle the root causes of allergy and intolerance, it is possible in many cases to reduce a child's long-term allergic potential and address any ongoing symptoms at the same time. My recipes, all specially created for this book, address some of the most common food allergens with notes on adapting the recipes to suit your child's needs. I have aimed for simplicity, using ingredients regularly found in supermarkets and health shops, and focusing on flavour profiles and combinations that are well placed to become family-friendly favourites. Whether you are a nervous or a competent cook, you'll find these recipes easy to follow and create. And, apart from providing vital nutrients that are so easily lacking in an allergy-free diet, they also follow the general healthy eating principles of providing your family with dishes that are low in sugar and rich in an array of nutrients, vitamins and minerals.

No matter what stage of the journey you're at as you begin reading, I recommend taking time to read the earlier parts of the book as well as delving into the recipes. Improving your child's overall immune-system health requires an understanding of what's happening to his or her immune system to have created an allergy or intolerance in the first place. I hope that, even if you've already got a diagnosis under your belt, understanding what that diagnosis means, and even looking back at the very many symptoms that could have been signs something was wrong, will give you a greater understanding of food allergy and intolerance, and therefore a greater sensitivity and intuition about how to help get things straight.

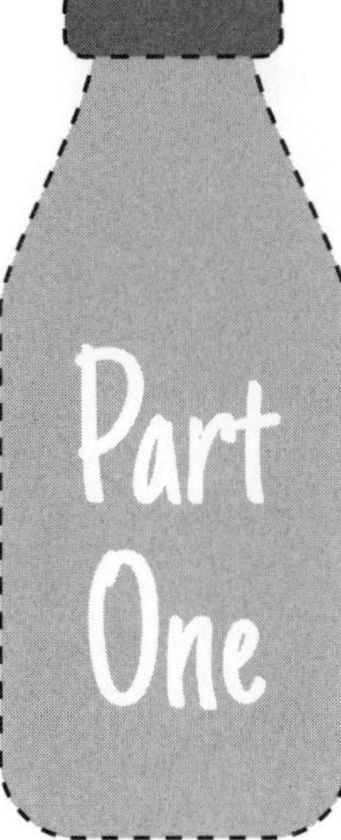

What does it all mean?

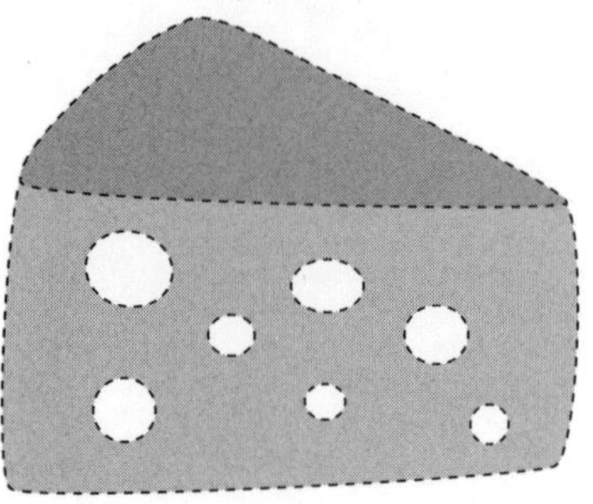

My approach to tackling food allergy in children is simple: to correct any imbalances in the body and facilitate the body's own healing process. However, before we can begin that journey, it's important to understand the nature of allergy – what it is, what it means, and what about your child brought you to this point and this book in the first place. Some of what follows you will already know – after all, I imagine you've come to this book because you've begun your food-allergy journey with your family – but in order to make sure we're all looking at things from the same position at the metaphorical dining table, it's important to recap.

You may find information here that you have had explained to you, but that you weren't sure about before. You may find information that makes you realize that the signs of food allergy in your child are more numerous than you first thought. Whatever stage you're at, I hope there's something here you can take away to shed light on where you are now in order that you can work together – as a family – to get things as on track as they can ever be.

Chapter 1

Where you are now

What's going on with my child?

Maybe you've noticed raised red spots on your son's skin after he's eaten certain foods. Perhaps your toddler constantly suffers with glue ear or sinusitis. Maybe you hear your daughter sneezing or sounding wheezy after certain meals. Perhaps you've noticed that while other kids settle down to some quiet time after supper, certain foods send your child into a frenzy. Perhaps you've noticed your teenager struggling with tummy pains and migraines for no apparent reason.

What do all these symptoms have in common? They are frequently caused by adverse food reactions. While some food reactions are immediate and dramatic (see box, page 11), many others are more subtle. Often, symptoms appear to be completely unrelated to anything to do with food (who would have thought glue ear might be food-related?) and it can take a long time before a pattern of symptoms emerges that makes diet an obvious cause. Many children – and parents – will suffer with illness for months or even years before anyone realizes there's an underlying immunity imbalance at fault.

When I see clients it's often only by looking in detail at health history, current signs and symptoms, and potential triggers that we identify a connection with diet. One of the most telling signs that food could be the cause of your child's suffering is if things dramatically improve during holidays, particularly holidays abroad, when we often eat differently to how we eat at home. Even a break from school meals can present a change in wellbeing that – now you think about it – could have been a sign.

Before we go any further, here are some telltale signs of food allergy or intolerance that you may have already noticed (it can be reassuring to know that these aren't necessarily out of the ordinary for children with food-related illness), or that may have cropped up without you even realising they were related. Of course, not every sign every time is a symptom of a food allergy or intolerance (after all, sometimes constipation, for example, is just the result of a diet lacking fibre or water), but when several symptoms appear together, frequently and consistently, they may be an indication that something is going wrong with your child's gut and immune response. At least, they are an indication that your child's reactions to food are worth investigating.

Skin reactions: Dry, flaky skin ✤ Eczema ✤ Itchy red skin ✤ Psoriasis ✤ Rashes and hives

Digestive symptoms: Bed wetting ✤ Bloated or swollen stomach ✤ Colic ✤ Constipation ✤ Diarrhoea ✤ Flatulence ✤ Irritable Bowel Syndrome (IBS) ✤ Mouth ulcers ✤ Poor appetite ✤ Poor growth ✤ Sleepiness after eating ✤ Stomach pains ✤ Vomiting

Other physical symptoms: Aches and pains in joints and muscles ✤ Anaphylaxis (see box, page 11) ✤ Breathing problems, wheezing, asthma ✤ Catarrh, mucus, sinus problems ✤ Ear, nose and throat infections ✤ Fatigue ✤ Headaches and migraines

Mental and emotional symptoms: Anxiety ✤ Attention Deficit Hyperactive Disorder (ADHD) ✤ Depression ✤ Food cravings ✤ Hyperactivity ✤ Irritability ✤ Loss of concentration, brain fog

✤ Sleep disorders (such as nightmares or night terrors, or frequent night waking)

There are further, more specific reactions that may occur depending upon the type of food allergy or intolerance your child experiences. We'll look at those in more detail later on.

What is anaphylaxis?

Anaphylaxis is a severe – potentially life-threatening – allergic reaction. If your child has trouble breathing or swallowing after eating something, it is essential you seek emergency medical help immediately.

Signs of anaphylaxis include:

- Chest pain
- Confusion
- Fainting, unconsciousness
- Shortness of breath, wheezing
- Swelling of the lips, tongue, throat
- Trouble swallowing
- Turning blue
- Weak pulse

Typically, children who are at risk of anaphylaxis in response to an allergen (whether that's food or anything else), will be given an epinephrine (adrenaline) auto-injector (often called an epi-pen) to carry with them at all times.

Your child's diagnosis

If you've picked up this book, you've probably already been through the process of testing and diagnosing your child's allergy. For some, having a label for the condition is a welcome relief – many parents I see tell me that they have had a long and frustrating journey to get to the point of understanding what their child's symptoms mean. At the same time, however, the slow realization of what a food allergy might mean, not only for your child but for the whole family, can soon become overwhelming. I want to reassure you that no matter how you're feeling right now, diagnosis is good news. It means you can start to equip your family for dietary and lifestyle changes that help tackle digestive problems for any and all of you head on.

Putting things in perspective

Getting to grips with a new diet and learning how to deal with everyday eating situations (at nursery, school or in restaurants), not to mention special occasions (birthday parties, holidays, family celebrations), pretty quickly makes us realize how so much of our lives – and the celebration of it – revolves around food. All of my children – three boys – suffer with food allergies. My own experience means I have witnessed first hand the many challenges parents of children with food allergies face, every day. But, despite my children's dietary restrictions, I have learned that an exciting, healthy and varied diet awaits every child no matter what their situation. I know that what once seemed daunting and unmanageable, with a few top tips and – most importantly – improved understanding, each allergy or intolerance affecting my boys was, in fact, an opportunity to explore a world of food far greater and more diverse and interesting than the one I might have otherwise provided for them.

Most importantly, I have learned that to support my boys' long-term health, to reduce the risk of any of them developing further allergies or intolerances, and to mitigate as many of their current symptoms as possible, I need to address the underlying causes of their food reactions – the imbalances in their bodies that were causing their immune systems to respond abnormally to food. Of course, the diagnosis you're given – the type of allergy your child has – is crucial. Some types of allergy are for life and, truthfully, it isn't always possible to overcome them, but that doesn't mean that nothing can be done at all. In some cases, you can desensitize a child's reactions to certain foods by creating a healthier gut and a better sense of balance throughout the body, and so alleviate symptoms. For less severe types of allergy, you may even enable the body to tolerate previous allergen foods again.

Chapter 2

Decoding allergies, sensitivities and intolerances

An allergen is any harmless substance that the body interprets (wrongly) as a pathogen, something harmful to health. This sets in motion a physical response intended to rid the body of the pathogen or protect against it. Allergens appear in many guises: in the foods we eat, the air we breathe, the pets we live with, and the chemicals, lotions, potions and medications we use in, on and around our body – to name a few.

Understanding the lingo

Rather confusingly, people often use the words allergy, sensitivity and intolerance interchangeably. However, each means something distinct and different from the others. To make matters more complicated, food reactions – even when they fall under the same umbrella term – can vary tremendously from one person to another. Think of it this way: just as one child's experience of a cold is not identical to another's, so each child's experience of a food reaction has its own, unique traits. This is particularly true when a reaction is delayed and the symptoms diverse, emerging over several months or even years, making diagnosis really tricky.

Food allergy in numbers

One of the most important messages you can take away with you at this early stage of the book is that if your child suffers with any type of food reaction, you are not alone. The latest surveys estimate that true food allergies affect up to 8 percent of children (while about 40 percent of British children suffer from one or more types of allergy, including non-food allergies). These account for between 20 and 50 percent of all cases of anaphylaxis (see box, page 11), resulting in food-allergy related deaths of between 150 and 200 people (children and adults) every year. This is six or seven times more fatalities than deaths resulting from reactions to insect stings. The number of children suffering severe nut or other food allergies has tripled in the last ten years.

Between 1997 and 2007, the number of reported cases of food allergy in children increased by 18 percent. In a similar timeframe, peanut allergy more than tripled in those under the age of 18 years – going from 0.4 percent in 1997 to 1.4 percent in 2008.

These figures do not, however, include those with food sensitivities and intolerances – which are thought to affect many, many more children and can often remain undiagnosed. Then, there are those diagnosed with coeliac disease, a gluten-related autoimmune condition (gluten is a protein found in wheat, barley and rye). Coeliac disease affects 1 in 100 people in the UK, although research suggests around 500,000 people remain undiagnosed.

The differences between each food reaction stem from the underlying mechanisms involved. Although you've probably already received your child's diagnosis, it can be helpful to understand how and why each type of food reaction occurs and what causes each specific set of symptoms. When you know why something happens, you can start to address the underlying imbalances in your child that may be contributing factors.

The role of the immune system

One of the easiest ways to describe what is happening during an allergic reaction is to imagine a cup that is half-filled with water. The cup is your child's immune system and the water is everything your child is exposed to in a healthy environment. The problem is that modern life adds extra water – representing dust mites, pet dander, pollen, ragweed, mould, environmental chemicals, medications, allergen foods and so on. Soon, the cup starts to overflow and the immune system is overloaded. It can't keep everything in check and so reacts to things that previously it considered harmless. This is why some children develop allergies as they grow, rather than being born with them.

The immune system is incredibly complex. It is designed to protect us from bacteria, viruses, parasites and anything else that threatens our wellbeing. Normally, it is brilliantly efficient at telling the difference between something that is harmless and something that is not (a pathogen – viruses and harmful bacteria, for example). Allergies occur when the immune system misreads a harmless substance, such as a food, as pathogenic and launches an antibody attack to destroy it (see box, opposite). Sometimes the immune system gets really confused and launches an attack against its own cells. When this happens we are said to have an autoimmune reaction (coeliac disease is an autoimmune condition as it causes the body to attack the delicate lining of the gut; see page 31).

Different types of food allergy trigger different types of immune response. In order to properly understand what's going on with your own child's immune response (and so how best to redress the balance to minimize its effects), it's important to understand what type of food allergy he or she has.

What is an antibody?

An antibody is a protein molecule that plays an important role in fighting against disease-causing viruses and bacteria. An antibody binds to a specific target (known as the antigen) and by doing so alerts components of the immune system to attack the culprit. In turn, the immune system produces a number of chemicals that promote an inflammatory response that effectively signals to other parts of the immune system to get to work. This inflammation also results in the symptoms of allergy.

The human body has several different classes of antibody – IgA, IgD, IgE, IgG and IgM – and they are involved in different aspects of our immune response. "Ig" stands for immunoglobulin, which is really just another name for an antibody. The letters A, D, E, G and M refer to the particular type of antibody, each one being primarily responsible for an immune response in a particular part or parts of the body or by a particular type of potential invader, and each one with its own special properties. They are like the body's five superheroes, each having its own special powers.

The different types of food reaction

So, we know that in simple terms a food allergy is an overreaction of the immune system to a food that in non-allergic people is harmless. However, we also know that the term "food allergy" is used interchangeably with other types of food reaction that may or may not involve the immune system at all. The main types I'll describe here are:

- True food allergies, which are subcategorized as IgE-mediated or non-IgE-mediated food allergy
- Food sensitivities
- Food intolerances
- Coeliac disease

IgE-mediated food allergy

When doctors refer to a food allergy, most of the time they are referring to an IgE-mediated food allergy, which you may also hear called a "true" or "classic" food allergy. Key features of an IgE-mediated food allergy are:

- It is most common in children, and rare in adults.
- Its symptoms tend to be immediate, typically occurring within two hours of eating and are normally very obvious.
- It can be triggered by consumption of only a tiny amount of food.
- The reactions it causes produce vast quantities of inflammatory chemicals such as histamine.
- It may result in a range of symptoms (see below), including itchy rashes, sneezing and in some cases anaphylaxis (see box, page 11).

- It is often self-diagnosed (because the reaction it causes is so obvious), although it can also be diagnosed through a skin-prick test or blood test.

The nature of an IgE-mediated food allergy

IgE-mediated food allergies usually run in families, so sometimes you'll be able to find a genetic link. Whether genetic or not, though, these allergies are a sign of underlying immune-system imbalance. Children who are prone to IgE-mediated reactions are said to have atopic syndrome (or to be hyperallergic) and may also have related conditions such as eczema, asthma and allergic rhinitis. Sometimes the related condition will show first; sometimes the food reaction.

Almost any food could be a culprit food for a child with an IgE-mediated food allergy. However, the most common IgE allergens in childhood are:

- cow's milk
- eggs
- fish and shellfish
- peanuts
- soybeans (and related products)
- tree nuts (e.g. almonds, pistachios, hazelnuts, walnuts, cashews, pecans, Brazils, macadamia nuts)
- wheat

Symptoms of an IgE-mediated food allergy

Typically, the first symptoms of an IgE-mediated food reaction occur around the mouth. This may include tingling, itching and swelling of the lips or tongue. Toddlers may scratch their ears or necks as they try to identify the source of the discomfort. It's really important to note that the reaction can result in swelling of the face and difficulty swallowing or breathing. For many children, though, the reactions don't stop there, and may go on to affect the whole body. For example, your child may experience:

- all-over itching
- a metallic taste in the mouth
- an all-over red rash (which may look like hives, urticaria or nettle rash)
- wheezing, choking, breathlessness
- repetitive coughing
- difficulty speaking or swallowing
- all-over puffiness (oedema)
- itchy, red and sore eyes and nose
- a flushed appearance
- a faster heartbeat and general feelings of anxiety or dizziness
- stomach pains, vomiting or nausea, diarrhoea or bladder incontinence

Some of these symptoms are obvious to a watchful parent, of course, but others rely on a child being able to describe how he or she is feeling. Children may say something like: "There's something stuck in my throat," "My tongue is too big," "My mouth itches," "Everything is spinning." You know your child best – remember to stay alert to comments that seem out of the ordinary, and take seriously any comment or sign that he or she is having trouble breathing. Shortness of breath requires immediate medical attention.

Living with an IgE-mediated food allergy

If your child is diagnosed with an IgE-mediated food allergy, you'll need to remember that even a small amount of culprit food can trigger a reaction, which means that you'll need to eliminate that food (or foods) completely from your child's diet, as well as take vigilant steps to avoid cross-contamination (see pages 136–56). Often families who have a child with an IgE-mediated food allergy decide to remove the culprit food from the house entirely, including removing it from the diet of other family members. Supporting the immune system through dietary measures can be helpful in the long term. If your child's reaction is likely to be severe, he or she may have to carry an auto-injector (see page 11).

Non-IgE-mediated food allergy

Exactly as its name suggests, this type of food allergy does not seem to involve IgE. Instead, it displays complex characteristics that include:

- Conditions such as eosinophilic gastroenteritis, coeliac disease (see page 30) and atopic eczema.
- In many cases, the need for greater quantities of the culprit food before a reaction takes place.
- Delayed reaction – symptoms may take 1–2 days to appear.
- Uncertainty as to which are the trigger food or foods (because the symptoms take longer to appear).
- Reactions triggered by the production of T-cells, immune cells that cause the body to produce various inflammatory chemicals that may affect any part of the body, but particularly affect the skin, respiratory system and digestive system.

The nature of a non-IgE-mediated food allergy can make it very difficult to diagnose. Usually, your child will have to try an elimination diet – removing possible culprit foods one by one and reintroducing them several weeks later to see if a reaction occurs.

IgE-mediated food allergy FAQs

There are lots of questions I'm often asked by families whose children are newly diagnosed with an IgE-mediated food allergy. Answering them all could take a book in itself, but here are the three most common questions I hear and the answers I give.

Raw and cooked foods – is there a difference?
Some allergens (for example, those found in fruits and vegetables) cause allergic reactions primarily when they are eaten raw. However, it is a mistake to think that cooking solves the problem, as most cooked culprit foods will still lead to a reaction of some description once they have made their way into the gut. So it is important to remove the culprit foods entirely from your child's diet, in whatever form they come.

My doctor says that my child may react to other, similar foods, too – is that right?
In some cases, yes. The phenomenon is known as cross-reactivity and it occurs when an antibody reacts not only to the original allergen, but also to a similar allergen, often one that shares similar structural composition or amino acids (the compounds that form the structure of a molecule) with the culprit food. For example, cross-reactivity is common among different shellfish, and among different

tree nuts. In some cases, including a condition known as oral allergy syndrome, cross-reactivity can occur when a child is exposed to the pollen from a plant with similar properties to the one that produces the culprit food. For example, if your child is allergic to apples or pears, he or she may also react to birch pollen.

Will my child grow out of his or her food allergy?

If your child has been diagnosed with a food allergy, only time will tell. About 80 percent of children grow out of milk and egg allergies, but only 20 percent tend to grow out of a peanut allergy. The best thing you can do for your child is follow medical advice as soon as the allergy is diagnosed, and then work towards balancing your child's immune system, supporting your child's body to minimize symptoms and give it the best possible chance of overcoming the allergy altogether, in time.

Once you've established the culprit food or foods, the safest way to treat this kind of allergy is to avoid those foods altogether. Children with a non-IgE-mediated food allergy are unlikely to need to carry an auto-injector (see page 11), as anaphylaxis is rare. However, creating a diet that supports the health of your child's gut is crucial.

Food sensitivity

A food sensitivity may or may not involve the immune system. In some cases, a food sensitivity involves immunoglobulins other than IgEs, such as IgG antibodies. It is estimated that up to

45 percent of people may suffer with food sensitivities, somewhat more than IgE-mediated food allergies, but they are often harder to identify.

- Reactions tend to be delayed, in some cases taking between one and two days to appear.
- Symptoms are varied, and may affect many different body systems, but they are not normally life-threatening.
- Reactions can be linked to other conditions, such as eczema, asthma, arthritis, migraines, ear infections, sinusitis and urticaria.
- Any food is a potential culprit for a food sensitivity – often, common everyday foods eaten in large quantities are most likely to trigger a reaction.

Non-coeliac gluten sensitivity is one common example of a food sensitivity, and is usually what people mean when they say they are reacting to gluten (but not suffering from coeliac disease).

Symptoms of food sensitivity

The list of symptoms associated with food sensitivity is long and varied, making it very hard to diagnose, especially when reactions are slow to emerge. If your child suffers from a combination of any of the following, frequently and in particular after eating certain foods, food sensitivity could be the problem.

- Allergic rhinitis, sinus problems, and repeated infections in the ears and throat
- Anxiety, depression, irritability
- Asthma
- Bed-wetting
- Constipation

- Eczema and other skin reactions
- Headaches, migraines
- Hyperactivity and behavioural problems
- Fatigue and sleep problems
- IBS symptoms, tummy pain
- Joint pain

Your doctor may have advised you to put your child on an elimination diet in order to pinpoint his or her culprit foods. In some cases, your child may be offered an IgG blood test.

Living with a food sensitivity

Very often, children experience more than one food sensitivity at a time, which can indicate general underlying digestive and immune-system imbalance. The first thing to do is to avoid the culprit foods in your child's diet for between three and six months. During this time you'll need to take positive steps to rebalance your child's immune system and provide a diet that helps to heal the digestive tract and improve gut health. After this period, if your child's symptoms have improved, and if your doctor and nutritionist agree, you can start to reintroduce culprit foods and monitor your child for any reactions. Bear in mind, though, that even if your child appears not to react to a food he or she was once sensitive to, you should avoid the temptation to offer it in large amounts. It is better to keep rotating it in the diet, to reduce the likelihood of that particular food becoming a problem again.

Food intolerance

Food intolerances are more common than food allergies, and less complex than food sensitivities. The main difference between a

Packaged-up food intolerances

Intolerance to lactose (a naturally occurring sugar found in milk and other dairy products) is the most common food intolerance worldwide, although generally it is more common in adults than in children (see page 28). Other common intolerance foods are those containing fructose (a fruit sugar found not only in fresh fruits, but also honey, corn syrup and many processed foods) and certain food additives (monosodium glutamate, sulphites and certain colourings among them). In fact, food additives are particularly problematic for young children, whose sensitive guts are less able to break down these chemicals.

Sulphites: Many foods are treated with sulphur dioxide in order to preserve their shelf life. You'll find them on food labels as sulphites and metabisulphites. The more packaged foods or processed foods your child consumes, the greater the number of chemical additives he or she will be ingesting into the body's system. I can never stress enough how important it is to cook from scratch whenever you can. I know that life is hectic for most families, and weekdays are often too busy for making a fresh meal every day – consider batch cooking at the weekends and freezing meals so that you have your own homemade ready-meal stash for the week. Know that every meal your child eats that avoids processed or packaged foods is a step closer to improved gut health. (It's also worth knowing that sulphite reactions have been shown to aggravate respiratory conditions, such as asthma.)

Monosodium glutamate (MSG): A flavour enhancer perhaps known best for its presence in takeaway Chinese foods, MSG is often an ingredient in tinned or packaged foods. It often produces very distinct sensitivity symptoms, including nausea, vomiting, headaches and dizziness. As with sulphites – cooking as many meals as possible from scratch is the surest way to protect your family from its harmful effects.

food intolerance and a food allergy is that a food intolerance does not involve the immune system and isn't life-threatening. If your child has been diagnosed with a food intolerance, you'll probably have achieved that diagnosis by working through an elimination diet, although lactose and fructose intolerance can be diagnosed via breath test.

A child develops a food intolerance when something in a food irritates his or her digestive system or when he or she is unable to properly digest – or break down – the food. As these reactions involve the digestive system many of the symptoms are linked to gut health. (This is another distinction from a food allergy, which can affect any part of the body.) Common digestive symptoms of food intolerance include the production of gas, bloating, abdominal pain and irregular bowel movements (particularly bouts of diarrhoea). Hives, urticaria, eczema and asthma are also symptoms associated with food intolerance, particularly an intolerance triggered by chemical food additives (see box, above).

Lactose intolerance

Lactose intolerance is not the same as a milk allergy and does not involve the immune system. Milk sugar (called lactose) consists of two sugar molecules – glucose and galactose – that are bound together. Lactose intolerance occurs when our body makes insufficient lactase enzyme, and so fails to split apart the two component sugars so that they can be properly absorbed in the small intestine.

At birth, most of us can produce lactase, which helps to digest and absorb the goodness from our mother's milk. However, as we grow, the body's production of this enzyme naturally starts to decrease. It's thought that a whopping 80 percent of the world's population starts to experience varying degrees of lactose intolerance as we mature into adulthood. Lactose intolerance is therefore more common in adults than children; while dairy allergies are more common in children. Certain ethnic groups are particularly at risk: 90 percent of Asian and 80 percent of black or Hispanic people report lactose intolerance symptoms. Gut infections, coeliac disease, inflammatory bowel diseases (such as Crohn's and colitis) are also risk factors. In such cases, once the underlying condition has been treated, many people find they can tolerate lactose again.

Symptoms of lactose intolerance in children, which typically occur between 30 minutes and 2 hours after consuming milk or milk products, are:

- bloating
- cramping, wind, or colic symptoms in babies
- nausea and diarrhoea

The easiest way to discover if lactose is causing your child's ongoing symptoms is to remove lactose-containing foods from his or her diet for two weeks. If symptoms improve after this time, ask your child to drink a glass of milk and monitor to see whether any of the symptoms recur. Alternatively, you can ask your doctor to give your child a lactose breath test (see page 36).

Lactose foods to avoid: Not all dairy foods contain high levels of lactose. Some (such as hard cheese and butter) contain levels low enough that children with only a mild intolerance are likely to be able to eat or drink them in small amounts.

Cow's milk, evaporated milk and condensed milk are the most concentrated sources of lactose. Foods that contain ingredients such as powdered milk, whey (the liquid remaining after milk has been curdled and strained) and whey protein concentrate may also be high in lactose. Some other examples of high-lactose foods include ice cream, soft-serve frozen yogurt, ricotta cheese, protein powders, energy bars, custard, and dulce de leche.

Cultured or fermented dairy products, such as cheese and regular yogurt, contain lower amounts of lactose, because the culturing process pre-digests much of the lactose. In addition, during the cheese-making process, as whey is removed, so is the lactose. Hard, aged cheeses are among the lowest lactose dairy foods. These include Cheddar, Parmesan, Swiss and other "block" cheeses. Furthermore, some manufacturers add lactase enzyme to certain dairy foods, such as some yogurts, to make them "lactose free".

Remember to look out for "hidden" sources of lactose, including baked goods such as breads, waffles and pancakes, as well as salad dressings, crisps, and margarine. Lactose is also sometimes added as a processing aid in the production of processed meats, including bacon, hot dogs and deli meats.

Living with a food intolerance

In most cases of food intolerance, the less of the culprit food your child eats, the fewer symptoms he or she will experience. Unlike with IgE-mediated food allergy, you won't necessarily have to eliminate the culprit food or foods from your child's diet in order to keep your child healthy. For example, some dairy products contain only traces of lactose and are, in most cases, perfectly safe for a child with a lactose intolerance to eat (check with your doctor or dietician first). Your child's digestive system is where his or her problems lie, so I strongly recommend you include foods in his or her diet to nourish and heal the gut and improve digestive function, while keeping culprit foods to a minimum. Also consider whether a gut infection or even coeliac disease may be exacerbating the problems your child is having. If you are concerned, ask your medical practitioner to help you get to the bottom of what's going on. In some cases, digestive enzyme supplements can be helpful to reduce symptoms.

Coeliac disease

Although it is often included with non-IgE-mediated food allergies, coeliac disease is specifically an autoimmune condition that, in genetically susceptible individuals, is triggered by eating gluten. It is one of the most chronic digestive disorders worldwide, affecting about 1 percent of the world's population and occurring in children and adults alike. Studies show that it is increasing in prevalence, with a sharp rise in diagnosis over the last two to three decades. In fact, over the last 50 years, coeliac disease incidences have increased by 400 percent.

Partly this is because we are increasingly aware of our health and better able to diagnose the disease. Nonetheless, experts anticipate that three-quarters of sufferers remain undiagnosed. Why? Because coeliac disease often presents no digestive symptoms at all.

If you or another member of your child's family has coeliac disease, your child's risk of developing the disease is estimated to be between 8 and 15 percent. It is also commonly associated with other autoimmune conditions, such as type-I diabetes and Hashimoto's disease (an autoimmune thyroid condition that leads to hypothyroidism).

Understanding coeliac disease

Autoimmune conditions are those where an overactive immune system attacks the body's own cells as if they were pathogens. In coeliac disease, the trigger for that autoimmune response is gluten, which sets off a chain reaction that causes the immune system to attack the delicate villi, tiny finger-like projections that line the small intestine and help with the gut's absorption and digestion of food. Those with coeliac disease produce antibodies that, in combination with other chemicals in the body, attack the intestine and flatten the villi, leading to malabsorption of nutrients and long-term illness. A child with coeliac disease may be low in certain vitamins and minerals as a result.

Although we know that coeliac disease is a genetically linked condition, having inherited the genes is not enough to develop the disease. In order to develop coeliac disease, a child (or any person) must have three things. First, he or she must have a genetic susceptibility to the disease. Second, he or she must eat gluten. And third, partially digested gluten products need to have got inside the cells of the gut lining, and into the blood stream, to set off the immune response. The last step involves the development of intestinal permeability, often referred to as leaky gut.

The symptoms of coeliac disease

The classic digestive symptoms of coeliac disease include abdominal pain, constipation, diarrhoea and bloating – symptoms that mean it can be misdiagnosed as irritable bowel syndrome (IBS). However, not all children with coeliac disease will have digestive symptoms. Coeliac disease can also affect the nervous system, the pancreas and other organs, including the gall bladder, liver and spleen. It has been linked to neurological problems, such as migraines, headaches, depression, attention deficit hyperactivity disorder (ADHD), autism and recurrent seizures (epilepsy). In adults, it may lead to increased risk of osteoporosis and, in adult women, to increased risk of miscarriage and infertility.

Babies with coeliac disease often have vomiting, abdominal distension or sudden changes in bowel movements – often alternating diarrhoea and constipation. They may appear generally run down and irritable. In toddlers it can lead to poor growth, little appetite, and ongoing stomach pains. In other cases, your dentist may comment on discolouration of teeth, poor dental enamel and the presence of mouth ulcers. Older children may exhibit short stature, behavioural problems, learning disabilities, autism, moodiness and depression, skin problems, or delayed puberty. Girls may have menstrual problems, such as delayed onset of menstruation, irregular periods, or even periods that start, then stop altogether. Your child may also complain of being tired all the time – this is often the result of malabsorption leading to low iron levels.

What does this mean for my child?

If your child has been diagnosed with coeliac disease, it is essential he or she follows a gluten-free diet for life (you must wait for a diagnosis before removing gluten, though). Even small amounts of gluten can damage the body and provoke ongoing symptoms.

You'll need to take extra care to avoid cross-contamination (see pages 136–56) and ensure your child's diet is truly, 100-percent gluten free.

In some cases (a warning sign should be if your child's health doesn't improve once you've removed gluten), cross-reactivity can also become a problem. Other foods, typically dairy, yeast-containing foods, oats, rice and corn, have been shown to cross-react with gluten and in some cases may also need to be removed from your child's diet. Blood tests are available to identify potential cross-reactive foods.

Interrelated allergic conditions

The human body is a complex system of interconnected biological and physiological processes. Inevitably, susceptibility to one type of allergy, disease or intolerance means that your child is likely to be more susceptible to other conditions, even if at first glance they seem unrelated. For example, studies show that 40 percent of children with moderate to severe eczema also have a food allergy, most commonly to egg. Food allergies have also been found to be a risk factor for asthma and allergic rhinitis (hay fever). You may find that other types of allergen – from the environment or from pets, for example – aggravate your child's food reactions, which can explain why removing culprit foods isn't always the final answer to improving symptoms.

It is also possible that children can have more than one type of food reaction. For example, children diagnosed with coeliac disease are often also lactose intolerant. This is because the enzyme lactase is produced in the villi, which are damaged in coeliac disease. As the villi recover and the gut heals, you may find your child can tolerate lactose again.

Coeliac disease and your child's skin

The genetic make-up that can lead to coeliac disease is also linked to a skin condition known as dermatitis herpetiformis, which can occur anywhere on the body and affects about 5 percent of people who suffer from coeliac disease. This is an incredibly itchy, blistering, angry-looking rash that many people easily mistake for eczema. The blisters can weep and become infected with the bacteria *Staphylococcus aureus*. Eliminating all gluten from your child's diet should help to clear up the rash.

Whatever diagnosis you've been given for your child, getting to the root cause of the allergy and treating underlying imbalances in his or her gut health and immune system will set your child on the path to long-term wellness, and perhaps even enable him or her to overcome the reaction altogether.

Testing and diagnosis

If you have picked up this book because you suspect your child has an allergy, and you don't yet have a diagnosis, it is important you seek professional support as soon as possible. A doctor, healthcare practitioner or allergy specialist will typically use both laboratory tests and elimination diets to find out what's going on in order to cover not only immediate food reactions, but those that can occur several days after eating a culprit food, too.

IgE testing

IgE-mediated food allergy is usually obvious because the reaction occurs very quickly after eating the culprit food. Nonetheless, your medical practitioner will confirm the diagnosis via a skin-prick or blood test. Once diagnosed you may be referred to an allergy specialist or dietician to advise you on medications and dietary changes. Allergy testing isn't an exact science and false positives, even false negatives, are possible. It's important to note that neither skin-prick nor blood tests will predict the severity of any potential allergic reaction.

Non-IgE and IgG testing

Looking for non-IgE and IgG food reactions can be a lengthy process, because the most common way to get to the bottom of what might be causing the problem is via an elimination diet. An alternative to an elimination diet, though, is a blood test (your child will still need to be eating the foods for an accurate blood test) – such as IgG antibody enzyme-linked immunosorbent assay (ELISA) tests or Food Allergen Cellular Test (FACT) tests.

Testing for coeliac disease

Blood tests are the first step in a diagnosis of coeliac disease. A doctor will order one or more of a series of blood tests to measure your child's response to gluten. It is important to remain on a gluten-containing diet prior to testing in order to ensure an accurate result. Sometimes a doctor may recommend an upper gastrointestinal endoscopy to confirm a diagnosis, although this is not always undertaken for children. In addition, a doctor may undertake gene testing – looking for the DQ2/DQ8 genes that are associated with coeliac disease. However, it is important to note this does not diagnose coeliac disease itself, but tells you if your child carries the genes associated with the condition. This can be useful if other family members have already been diagnosed with coeliac disease, because it identifies risk. Normally, doctors will use a cheek swab, which is sent away for analysis. Unlike blood tests, genetic testing doesn't require your child to have been eating gluten during the diagnostic process.

If all the coeliac tests are negative for the disease, but you still suspect your child has a problem with gluten, your healthcare provider will probably recommend an elimination diet and/or a specific blood test for non-coeliac gluten sensitivity.

Food intolerance testing

The only ways to test for lactose and fructose intolerance are through (most likely) an elimination diet or (occasionally) a breath test. The breath test takes about two hours and measures

The elimination diet

Although any food protein has the potential to cause an allergic reaction, it is estimated that around eight to ten foods (fewer than the complete 14-strong allergen list issued by the UK's Food Standards Agency; see page 123) account for 90 percent of all food reactions. These foods are:

- cow's milk
- eggs
- peanuts
- fish

- shellfish, including crustacea, such as crab, lobster, crayfish, shrimp and prawn, and molluscs
- tree nuts (namely almonds, hazelnuts, walnuts, cashews, pecans, Brazils, pistachios, macadamia nuts)
- wheat and cereals containing gluten (wheat, barley, rye, regular oats)
- soybeans and related products

Other common offenders include sesame, citrus fruits, yeast, kiwi and corn, as well as additives.

The traditional way to identify problematic foods is to eliminate the suspect foods and monitor any change in symptoms in your child. There are many versions of an elimination diet – usually it means removing the commonly offending foods from your child's diet (along with aggravating foods, such as foods containing sugar, sweeteners, caffeine and additives) for about three weeks then reintroducing them one by one and monitoring reactions. Your healthcare provider will guide you through the process most suitable for your child's situation and symptoms. I recommend keeping a food diary throughout the process – note down every day what your child eats and drinks, even in tiny quantities, and also your child's symptoms, looking for behavioural symptoms and mood changes, as well as physical symptoms such as bloating and rashes.

If symptoms do not improve over the course of the elimination diet, your child may have other underlying conditions or imbalances, such as a gut infection, that are co-existing alongside his or her reactions to food.

the amount of hydrogen gas in your child's breath at 15-minute intervals during that time. The more hydrogen is present, the more likely there is an intolerance. Other suspected food reactions, such as to MSG or sulphites (see box, page 26), are more commonly identified by an elimination or "challenge" diet – your healthcare provider will encourage you to remove potentially reactive foods from your child's diet and monitor his or her symptoms. This is then followed by a "challenge" where the suspect foods are introduced and, again, symptoms are monitored.

Chapter 3

Allergy and immunity

If you're reading this book, the chances are you are already aware that your child has allergies. The good news is that there is much you can do not only to reduce the symptoms naturally, but also prevent other allergies developing. Not only that but by addressing the root causes of an allergic response, certain atopic conditions, such as eczema and food sensitivities, can be dramatically improved.

Before I discuss how you can reduce your child's allergic potential, let's look at why your child has developed a food reaction and what the risk factors are. For the sake of ease, in this chapter and in the remainder of the book, I'm going to refer to food reactions in general as "food allergies" unless I need specifically to refer to an allergy, sensitivity or intolerance, or to coeliac disease.

Why has my child developed a food allergy?

Allergies – food and otherwise – are on the rise in both children and adults. Why some people develop antibodies against certain foods is not fully understood. When it is working optimally, your child's immune system should spend most of its time in a state of observational inactivity. This means that *most of the time*, the job of the immune system is not to respond to what's going on in your child's environment and body, launching an attack only when something truly potentially harmful decides to invade.

Allergies in children are a clear sign that the immune system is out of balance – it is reacting when it shouldn't be. The good news is that your child's immune system is incredibly adaptable, which means that there are numerous opportunities – particularly during the early years of life – to positively influence immune response. So, while you can't change what's been going on historically, there is much you can do to influence your child's future immune-system health.

While certain food allergies can have a genetic link (see box, opposite), simply having a genetic predisposition to allergy does not predetermine your child's likelihood of developing that allergy at birth or beyond. There are many other factors that can influence allergic potential:

- levels of healthy bacteria (gut flora) in your child's intestine, and general gut health
- being born vaginally or by C-section
- being breastfed or bottle-fed
- time of weaning
- nutritional intake and diet quality
- exposure to environmental bacteria during childhood
- how often your child has certain medications, including antibiotics

Looking after your child's gut health

Our body is the dwelling place for about 100 trillion bacteria and other microbes, collectively known as our microbiome. The microbes fulfil many important jobs, including breaking down our food, making nutrients, fighting off infection and supporting our immune system. Did you know, in fact, that around 80 percent of your child's immune system lies within his or her gut

The genetics of food allergy

We cannot change our genes, but a child who has a genetic predisposition to something will not necessarily go on to develop the full-blown condition of that something. Rather, the interaction of your child's developing immune system with his or her environment influences the outcome. This is known as epigenetics. How we live – our nutrition, the toxins we're exposed to in our environment, and even the lifestyle of our ancestors – can influence whether certain genes activate in our own make-up (and in the make-up of our children). We carry an historical imprint of the lifestyles of all our ancestors, and we can influence that imprint in the way we live our own lives. As parents and carers, part of our responsibility is to provide a lifestyle and environment that creates the best possible permutation of "switched-on" genes in our children. Your influence over your child's allergy symptoms is very real, and if you are a biological parent was so even before your child was a twinkle in your eye.

in the form of friendly bacteria? In babies these friendly bacteria support the development of the immune system, teaching it the difference between microbial friend and foe. Through their work, the friendly bacteria teach the immune system not to react to certain harmless antigens, including food.

Our gut microbes have other good work to do, too. They produce various substances such as butyrate (see page 00) that nourish the gut and help calm down any inflammation in the digestive tract. They also help to maintain a healthy gut barrier and prevent leaky gut (see below). It is hardly surprising, then, that maintaining a healthy gut flora plays a crucial role in reducing the risk of allergies in children, and minimising symptoms in those who already have them. In fact, studies have shown that children with IgE-mediated food allergies tend to have a different gut flora from those who don't.

Imbalances in a child's gut flora can occur for many reasons. Poor diet, particularly one of excess sugar, processed foods and ready meals, and that lacks fruit and vegetables and fibre-rich and fermented foods is the first, and most easily influenced when we're looking after children. Antibiotics, and persistent exposure

Innate immunity and oral tolerance

Our fundamental, inborn immunity is known as the innate immune system. We all have it – it includes physical barriers such as our skin, as well as specific immunity cells that are found in our gut. Not only does it act as a baby's first line of defence against the pathogens he or she encounters when first thrust into the world, it also helps to develop something called oral tolerance. This is the name given to the immune system's ability to remain inert when we eat. In other words, oral tolerance prevents the immune system from reacting to food "foreign bodies" that are in fact harmless. When there is a breakdown in oral tolerance – perhaps because there is imbalance in a child's gut flora – food allergies and other reactive conditions may develop.

to environmental chemicals and toxins are also harmful to a child's (and anyone's) microbiome. As parents, providing a diet that is rich in fibre, fermented foods and probiotics (see page 00), reducing our children's consumption of sugar and processed foods, and avoiding antibiotics whenever it's safe to do so are the best ways to help our children develop a healthy gut microbiome. And don't forget that your children learn from you – eat healthily yourself and not only will that have a positive epigenetic effect on any children you have in the future, your example teaches the children you already have how to eat healthily.

Leaky gut

The health of your child's intestinal lining is vital not only to his or her overall health, but also to their risk of developing food allergies. Our gut is lined with millions of epithelial cells that are responsible for maintaining a barrier between our gut contents (the intestinal lumen) and our blood stream. A healthy gut allows small nutrients to cross the gut barrier into the blood stream, and keeps back large food proteins. However, when the intestinal barrier becomes compromised (what we know as "leaky gut" syndrome), large dietary proteins make their way through the barrier, enter the blood, stimulate an immune response, and produce symptoms characteristic of various allergic diseases.

At birth, the gut lining is at its most permeable, which can make babies vulnerable to adverse immune reactions. This is one of the reasons why new mothers are encouraged to breastfeed: breast milk is rich in colostrum and immunoglobulins that make it particularly effective at sealing up the gut lining quickly.

Damage to the gut lining may occur for a variety of reasons: gut infections, overconsumption of certain foods (particularly gluten), lack of digestive enzymes, medications (such as

Pregnancy, birth and breastfeeding

Your child's immune system began developing even before he or she was born. During the later stages of pregnancy, good bacteria start to populate the unborn baby's gut. At vaginal birth, exposure to the mother's microbiome in the birth canal is believed to further this process, exposing the baby to bacteria that help prepare the immune system for learning the good from the bad (studies show that babies born by C-section may develop a different balance of gut flora to those born vaginally). Amazingly, new research suggests that the baby may even have its first exposure to the mother's microbiome while still in the womb, which means expectant mothers are now encouraged to improve their own gut flora during pregnancy. Eating fermented foods (such as yogurt, kefir and sauerkraut) and plenty of fibre, taking probiotics, and avoiding certain medications are all ways to do this.

Recent studies show that the development of oral tolerance before birth depends upon the interaction of gut microbes and the food fragments from the food the expectant mother consumes. In other words, what the mother eats or does not eat during pregnancy can be important. If an expectant mother deliberately avoids certain foods, such as peanuts for example, there is no opportunity for the foetus to develop oral tolerance. As long as the mother herself does not have a severe allergy to a certain food, women are now advised that including a wide range of foods during pregnancy, including common allergen foods in low doses, may be able to increase the baby's tolerance to them later in life.

Breastfeeding

Breast milk contains a diverse range of immune-modulating compounds and beneficial bacteria that can help shape a baby's immune system. Breast milk also contains prebiotics – compounds that support the growth and development of the baby's gut flora – and various other compounds that support the development of a healthy gut barrier (see page 56). The presence of IgA in breast milk helps prevent potential toxins from entering the baby's blood stream and we know that good levels of IgA help to develop oral tolerance. Newborn babies are temporarily deficient in their ability to produce IgA, making breast milk an important early source.

Finally, breastfed babies receive minute amounts of numerous food antigens from the foods the mother eats. This helps expose the baby to a wide range of different foods in very small doses, which can also help the baby develop oral tolerance.

For new mothers who are unable to breast feed, one option is to include mixed-strain probiotic supplements (containing *Lactobacillus* and *Bifidobacterium* and *Saccharomyces boulardii*) to formula milk. Various studies have found the use of certain probiotics in formula-fed babies can reduce the risk of the baby going on to develop allergies. These supplements are also suitable for expectant mothers during pregnancy and may help the baby even before birth.

antibiotics, non-steroidal anti-inflammatory drugs [NSAIDs] and steroid medications), stress, nutritional deficiencies (particularly of vitamins A and D and zinc) and excess sugar in the diet are among them. Premature birth, and weaning before the age of four months may also play a role.

Weaning and allergies

Weaning advice is always changing, so wherever you are in your child's development, the advice you were given when your child was a baby is now probably updated or modified in some way.

Weaning and coeliac disease

If you have a family history of coeliac disease, you may be wondering whether the timing of introducing gluten has any effect on the risk of your child developing coeliac disease. Studies are currently inconclusive: some suggest introducing gluten early (between four and six months) to reduce the risk of developing coeliac disease; others suggest it makes no difference at all. There are various risk factors associated with developing coeliac disease and it is thought that one of the reasons why coeliac disease has increased dramatically over the last 50 years may be owing to changes in our gut microbiome, as well as changes to our diet (increased gluten, sugar and processed foods). These influences cause an imbalance in our gut flora and therefore our immunity. So, supporting your child's gut health and microbiome may be just as important as when you introduce gluten.

The more we understand about the immune system in babies, the more we realize how we can influence its development with the timing and types of foods introduced during the weaning process. The most up-to-date research suggests that exposing a child to potentially allergenic foods (such as milk, wheat, gluten, nuts, peanuts and so on) early on in weaning may reduce the allergy risk. That does not mean a baby should be weaned before four months old, because the baby's immature or incomplete gut lining (see page 43) can mean that food particles cross into the blood stream, but weaning should start by six months, and can include tiny amounts of common allergens.

Of course, if your child has a high genetic risk of developing allergies (particularly classic IgE-mediated food allergies; see page 18), take advice from your GP or allergy consultant. You will probably need to take extra precautions.

Playing in the puddles

It seems strange to think that modern emphasis on protecting children from germs and keeping them clean may actually contribute to food allergies later in life. It's no coincidence that children who grow up on farms – surrounded by animals and mud – are known to be less prone to allergic conditions. All this is the basis of the hygiene hypothesis, which suggests that because of improved hygiene and vaccinations, our immune system comes into minimal contact with bacteria, viruses and parasites and doesn't learn how to tell whether there is a stranger or friend at the door. In its confusion, it starts to react to harmless antigens, such as food. Use of antibiotics, particularly early in life, has also been associated with an increased risk of developing allergies – the immune system misses the opportunity to learn to do the work properly itself.

During early childhood as your child's immune system is

developing and maturing, exposure to various microbes is helpful in promoting normal immunity development. Encourage your children to play outside, get dirty and play with other children. You may want to get a pet: children living with pets, particularly in the first few years of life, have been shown to have lower incidence of allergic disease.

Vitamin D and immunity

Population studies have shown that there is a discernible link between the risk of an individual developing a food allergy and levels of vitamin D in the blood. Furthermore, through observing the patterns of food allergy in children, scientists have hypothesized that the time of year a baby is born may have a bearing on how likely he or she is to develop a food allergy: various studies demonstrate a low proportion of food allergies in children born during the summer and spring months – when we have the most hours of sunshine, our main 'source' of vitamin D.

But, why is vitamin D so important? Vitamin D has both direct and indirect effects on the function of the cells of our immune system. For example, vitamin D can help the body to manufacture regulatory T-cells (known as Tregs), which can suppress inflammatory responses and promote allergen tolerance. Vitamin D also supports gut health, including promoting a healthy gut barrier, which we know is so important for a balanced immune system (see page 57).

The importance of key nutrients

A healthy immune system and digestive tract requires key nutrients, vitamins and minerals. Any deficiencies could compromise their function, which may increase the risk of developing food allergies. Vitamins A and D, essential fats and zinc are just some of the key nutrients that need to be at an optimum in your child's diet in order to ensure a balanced immune system. We'll look into how to ensure optimum nutrition in your family diet later in the book.

What is immunotherapy?

Allergen immunotherapy (AIT) has shown promising results in reducing the risk of life-threatening allergic reactions in people who are accidentally exposed to an allergen. It has been used effectively in the treatment of airborne allergens. However, food allergen immunotherapy is still currently under investigation to ensure that it is effective and safe for children with IgE food allergies.

The AIS technique aims to make the body less reactive to an allergenic food by giving the sufferer very small doses of the food daily, gradually increasing the amounts. This process is known as desensitization, and it must be maintained and monitored regularly in order to be effective. The doses are ingested (eaten), sublingual (under the tongue) or fixed (via applications on the skin). Studies so far have focused on cow's milk, hen's eggs and peanuts – all common childhood allergens – but it is a time-demanding procedure and is not suitable for all children. However, as more studies are done, it may become a promising treatment in the long term.

Chapter 4

Tackling allergies – getting to the root of the problem

So, how can we help our children find a long-term resolution to a food reaction? While conventional medicine can be very helpful, and in cases of severe IgE-mediated food allergy conventional medicine can be life-saving, it is not without its drawbacks. The conventional approach is usually to treat the symptoms and calm down the immune system with the use of antihistamines and other inflammatory-inhibiting medicines, decongestants and corticosteroids. In some cases, doctors may prescribe techniques such as subcutaneous immunotherapy – or allergy shots – where a child receives injections of very small amounts, in gradually increasing doses, of the offending substance(s) to promote desensitization.

But I believe it is possible to go beyond simply treating the symptoms of an allergy and in addition get to the root of the problem. Tackling underlying immune-system imbalances requires a functional nutritional approach that, for those with IgE-mediated food allergies and coeliac disease, can improve symptoms long term and reduce the risk of other allergies developing. As there are more children affected by food sensitivities and atopic conditions than true allergies, this approach can bring relief to many other children and families, too.

Your allergy-busting action plan

Having a step-by-step action plan to tackle the underlying imbalances in your child's immune system can help whatever allergies your child is facing. That does not necessarily mean they will be able to eat specific foods again, but it will help rebalance their immune-system response, nourish and repair any disrupted mucosal barriers (skin, lungs, gut and so on) and reduce the risk of developing further food reactions in the future. Here's how to tackle the root causes of food allergies:

- Reduce the allergen burden as much as possible.
- Calm the immune system to establish a more appropriate balance in the immune-system response, and reduce allergy symptoms.
- Restore and optimize the health of the digestive tract.

1. Reducing the allergy burden

Your first step is to remove all the known triggers involved in your child's allergies. This is not always as straightforward as it seems. While you may be aware of the IgE trigger foods affecting your child, there could be other food sensitivities that have remained hidden beneath the bigger problem. I frequently see clients whose children are suffering from reactions not only to the food they have identified as the culprit, but also other IgE foods, as well as IgG foods, gluten and additives, and even non-food related allergens such as pollen, dust, pet hairs, moulds or toxins. In some cases, a child will also need to avoid cross-reactive foods (see page 22). If you suspect there are other triggers, speak to your healthcare practitioner who may be able to undertake further testing or recommend an elimination diet. Once you know better what you're dealing with, avoid all those allergens as much as you can and according to each specific case. For example:

- If your child has IgE-mediated food allergies or coeliac disease, then he or she will need to eliminate the culprit foods completely and for life. While it is true that some children may grow out of certain IgE allergens, you should not re-introduce these foods unless you have medical advice and careful medical supervision.
- If your child has been diagnosed with IgG food sensitivities, he or she may be able to tolerate those foods in the future. The normal recommendation is to remove the culprit foods for between three and six months while you address any other imbalances (such as gut infections) and introduce a diet that supports gut healing.

2. Calming the immune system

It is important to consider other triggers that may disturb the immune system and so aggravate allergy symptoms. Childhood stress, for example, can upset the balance of gut flora and intensify all symptoms; while using antibiotics can change the balance of good bacteria in your child's gut. Take a look at your child's overall diet, too. Unprocessed, organic foods, low in sugars and refined carbohydrates are important to help calm the immune system and reduce inflammation. All the recipes in this book are designed to support the gut and the immune system, helping to nourish your child healthily to restore balance.

There are specific anti-allergy and anti-inflammatory foods and nutrients you can include in your child's diet. All the recipes in the book contain them in bucket-loads, but it's worth separating them out here, so that you can mix, match and create in your own ways, too.

Antioxidant-rich fruit and vegetables: Studies suggest a high intake of fruits and vegetables will support immunity and reduce the risk of allergies. Fruits and vegetables are packed with antioxidants and other nutrients that can help calm allergic symptoms. Among these are flavonoids, such as quercetin, vitamin C, vitamin A, sulphur compounds, and minerals such as magnesium. These can calm the body's systems and reduce the inflammatory response, which is a result of the immune system overreacting. Try to give your child at least five portions of vegetables every day and two to three portions of fruit. Aim for as much colour in the diet as possible and keep it varied.

Plant antioxidants quercetin and anthocyanins are found in many fruits and vegetables and are particularly beneficial as they help to stabilize mast cells, which are key components of the immune response and release histamine, a chemical often associated with allergic symptoms. Foods rich in quercetin include apples, berries, broccoli, cherries, citrus fruits, fennel, plums, red onions and spinach. Anthocyanin-containing foods include berries, cherries, grapes, red cabbage, red onion and wild rice. Antihistamine properties are also found in lots of herbs: chamomile, Holy Basil (tulsi), parsley and thyme among them. The wonderful thing about herbs is that they make a brilliant replacement for salt and other flavourings to make food really delicious and appealing for kids. Use liberally!

Good fats: Children are often susceptible to having low levels of polyunsaturated omega-3 essential fatty acids in their diet. These are good fats that, along with monounsaturated fats (found in foods such as avocado, olives and macadamias), are particularly important for reducing inflammation in the body, which in turn can help to reduce allergy symptoms. Good sources of omega-3 fats include oily fish (anchovies, herring, mackerel, salmon and sardines – try to include these in meals at least three times a week); chia seeds, flaxseeds, pumpkin seeds, walnuts and their oils in smoothies and dressings (but not for cooking); leafy greens and some algal sources (including spirulina powder, and sea vegetables, such as nori and dulse). Meat from wild or grass-fed animals and free-range or organic eggs can also contain omega-3 fats.

In contrast, saturated fats and omega-6 fatty acids in excess can promote inflammation. Avoid using large amounts of margarine, or corn, vegetable, sunflower and soybean oils. Processed foods are often high in saturated fats – an allergy-sensitive diet should avoid processed foods as much as possible.

Sugar-free: Sugary foods and drinks have an inflammatory effect in the body as well as being low in nutrients, so its time to ditch the sugar. This isn't just a warning against refined sugar, but also against unrefined sugar and includes syrups such as agave and maple syrup. The one exception is the inclusion of a little local raw honey, particularly if your child has seasonal allergies, such as hay fever (which commonly accompanies food allergy), as it may help to educate your child's immune system to tolerate local pollen.

Spices: Turmeric is one of the most effective natural remedies for allergies. Not only is turmeric root inexpensive (try mixing it into warm milk or milk alternative), it has many beneficial healing properties. Research shows that turmeric reduces inflammation and lowers histamine levels. It is also an effective decongestant, making it useful for nasal symptoms. Turmeric's primary active component is a compound called curcumin, a powerful antioxidant that is also available as a supplement. Try mixing a teaspoon of turmeric with a spoonful of local honey and offer it just as it is as a sweet treat, or mixed into fruit purée and yoghurt. Alternatively, simply add it to soups, curries, salad dressings, rice dishes and casseroles, or in warming drinks and teas. Try ginger, too – another natural anti-inflammatory. A good decongestant and antihistamine, ginger is delicious in juices, smoothies and all sorts of cooking.

Low-histamine foods: If your child is experiencing a flare up with their symptoms such as itchy skin, hives, sneezing, nasal congestion or headaches you may wish to avoid foods high in histamine, such as avocados, aged cheese, citrus fruits, cocoa, fish and shellfish, pickles and spinach to name a few, and stick to those that have low histamine levels, such as freshly cooked meat; poultry (frozen or fresh); freshly caught fish; eggs; gluten-free grains (quinoa, rice and so on); certain fresh fruits (including apples, cantaloupe melon, kiwis, grapes, mangoes, pears and watermelon), fresh vegetables (except aubergine, avocado, spinach and tomatoes); and dairy substitutes (such as almond milk, coconut milk, hemp milk, rice milk).

Using supplements

I always tell my clients that, while supplements are not a replacement for a nutritious diet, particularly when it comes to children, they can be a good way to help balance things out and restore equilibrium in a child who is suffering. When it comes to calming the immune system, supplements containing a concentrated source of anti-inflammatory and/or histamine-lowering nutrients are the ones to look out for. Some of the best supplements to consider are: boswellia, butterbur, curcumin, vitamin C, ginger, medicinal mushrooms (such as reishi), nettle, omega-3 fatty acids, quercetin, resolvins and spirulina.

In some children, a B-vitamin complex can help to lower histamine, while diamine oxidase (DAO) enzyme will also help to metabolize histamine and eliminate it from the body. Supplementing with digestive enzymes can play a role in reducing your child's allergic potential, relieve intolerances and improve overall digestive health, as can supplements of zinc.

Secretory immunoglobulin A (SIgA): SIgA coats the gut lining and is designed to protect us from pathogens and toxins. A persistently low level of SIgA can increase a child's risk of food allergies and leaky gut. Babies naturally have low levels of SIgA, although breast feeding can improve levels quickly. Low levels can be genetically linked, but other factors, including stress, gut imbalances, certain medications and low levels of key nutrients – particularly vitamin A – can also play a role. Supplements to improve levels include the probiotic yeast *Saccharomyces*

The magic of sulphur

MSM (methylsulfonylmethane) is a form of sulphur that is natural mineral component of many foods, including breast milk. Important for the health of our skin, immune system and gut, among other body systems, MSM appears to relieve allergies in a number of ways. It can reduce the symptoms of leaky gut. It can help reduce allergic symptoms, improve skin conditions, and reduce allergy-related pain, swelling and digestive symptoms. Available as a power supplement, MSM can be added to your children's smoothies or stirred into yogurt and stewed fruit.

boulardii (this isn't suitable if your child has a yeast allergy), probiotics, and vitamins A and D.

3. Healing and restoring the digestive tract

Some parents find that even with the avoidance of the known allergy foods, a child's allergy symptoms do not significantly improve. He or she might even experience ongoing digestive problems. One of the underlying reasons why some children show little improvement lies with fundamental imbalances in the digestive tract. With a little detective work, though, it is possible to identify the key gut imbalances and take steps to heal and restore a healthy gut.

Signs of gut imbalance

If, having removed all trigger foods and taken steps to calm the immune system, your child's symptoms have not improved, it is worth considering a gut imbalance to be at the root cause. The following are the telltale signs, although they may not always occur:

- abdominal bloating especially after eating, abdominal pain, or generally feeling that the tummy feels worse after eating
- excessive burping or flatulence, often odorous
- gastric reflux, which may be accompanied by a burning sensation in the chest
- constipation or diarrhoea, or alternating between the two
- nausea
- pale or "floating" stools

If your child is complaining of ongoing digestive symptoms such as these, he or she may have a gut infection. Unwanted bacteria, yeasts or parasites present in the gut can lead to changes in immune activity, inflammation and leaky gut, which (as we've already seen) in turn can increase the number of food reactions. They can also stimulate the production of histamine, which can result in allergic symptoms.

Gut infections are much more common than you may think. There are many ways children can pick up infections: not washing hands properly, having physical contact with infected children or adults, and eating improperly cooked or stored foods are among the most common. A diet high in sugar and carbohydrates or regular use of antibiotics can also lead to changes in our normal gut flora and enables harmful microbes to flourish or become problematic. It takes a comprehensive stool test to identify gut infections. You can arrange one of these for your child through a doctor, or a nutrition or healthcare practitioner.

If your child is diagnosed with a gut infection, it is important to work with a qualified practitioner to help eradicate it. Providing meals packed with natural antimicrobial foods (such as cloves, oregano, turmeric, olive oil and coconut oil), minimizing sugars (which encourage the growth of pathogens and promote inflammation), and reducing any constipation (see box, page 60) to help eliminate toxins and reduce bloating and tummy pain will also support conventional intervention and speed recovery.

Improving digestion

The process of digestion involves the body breaking down the food we eat in order that we can absorb key nutrients and expel the waste. If your child's body is not producing adequate levels of hydrochloric acid and digestive enzymes in order to do that job, it can increase the risk of food reactions. This is particularly noticeable in certain food intolerances. For example, a lactose intolerance suggests your child's body isn't producing sufficient amounts of the enzyme lactase to digest the lactose (milk sugar; see page 28).

When food is incompletely digested, large amounts of intact food molecules reach the gut wall, causing damage and inflammation which can contribute to leaky gut. These large food molecules may then cross the gut lining and enter the blood stream, resulting in an immune reaction. Incompletely digested food in the gut can also feed unwanted gut microbes. This can lead to fermentation in the gut which produces gas that leads to pain, bloating and flatulence, as well as nutrient malabsorption. Deficiency in zinc can particularly exacerbate the problem as it can affect digestive secretions and contribute to leaky gut. Try to include zinc-rich food in your child's diet, including seafood, beef, pork and chicken; spinach, mushrooms and sea vegetables; and pumpkin seeds, cashew nuts and raw cacao.

You can also naturally improve digestion by including enzyme-rich foods in your child's diet. These include fresh pineapple, papaya and sprouted seeds and beans. Fermented foods, such as kimchi and sauerkraut, apple cider vinegar, lemon juice and pickles can help stimulate digestive secretions. Bitter greens and sour foods (chicory, rocket (arugula), watercress, dandelion) and fresh turmeric, which can be added to soups and stews or added to salads, can also be effective digestive aids. Another trick is to use a slow cooker or slow cook dishes in the oven. The lengthened cooking process breaks down the tough collagen fibres in meat, producing a delicious, softer consistency, which is easier on the digestive tract.

Healing a leaky gut

If you've read this book from the beginning, you'll know by now that repairing any damage to your child's gut wall can be important to reduce the effects of food allergy. First and foremost it's important to remove all culprit foods from your child's diet.

Tackling constipation

Various studies have shown a link between food sensitivities (particularly to gluten and dairy) and constipation in children. However, constipation is one of the easiest things to deal with at home, through dietary and lifestyle adjustments.

Increase dietary fibre: The muscles of the walls of the small and large intestine require something to push against in order to maintain tone and proper function. This bulk is provided by fibre, a form of indigestible carbohydrate. Good sources of fibre are fresh fruit (papaya and kiwifruit are particularly good) and vegetables, prunes and stewed apple, gluten-free grains, oat bran, and nuts and seeds. A really good tip is to every day try adding 1 tablespoon of ground flaxseed to your child's breakfast, and then follow up by giving a glass of water to drink. Alternatively, try adding it to a homemade smoothie (smoothies are better than juices as they include the fibre part of the fruit and vegetables, too) or stir it into porridge or yogurt. For additional benefit, try adding ground flaxseed to prune juice, which can also stimulate bowel movements. For stubborn constipation in older children you can repeat the flaxseed remedy later in the day.

Encourage water: Fibre needs adequate amounts of water to form a soft stool. Encourage your child to take a water bottle to school and to sip it throughout the day. Most schools now have water fountains where children can top up their bottles when they run out, and many will even allow children to have water bottles with them during lessons. If constipation is a problem for your child, talk to his or her school about their drinking policy and discuss ways in which they can support your efforts to encourage your child to drink more.

Focus your supplements: Certain supplements are particularly good for encouraging bowel movements. **Magnesium**, for example, relaxes the muscles in the intestines, which helps to establish a smoother rhythm of intestinal contractions. It also attracts water, which increases the amount of water in the colon and softens the stool. **Vitamin C** (given in powdered form) is a natural laxative, again by encouraging water into the stool. Consult the packaging to make sure you're giving the right amount, although the only adverse affect will be loose stools. Finally, **probiotic** supplements that contain *Bifidobacterium lactis* (*B. lactis*) may shorten the time it takes for the stool to pass through your child's intestine.

Give the bowels time to do their thing: Don't rush your child if he or she needs a poo – even if you have somewhere you all need to be. It's thought that our stressed lifestyles are a major cause of constipation for all of us.

Make time for running around: Aerobic exercise can help to stimulate bowel movement. Give your child lots of opportunity to run around or take part in structured exercise daily.

Once you're all on track with that, you need to ensure that you give your child's gut lining optimal nourishment to help it heal and repair itself. There are are a range of key nutrients.

- **Vitamin A:** One of the most important vitamins for gut and immune system health, vitamin A is found naturally in eggs, full-fat dairy products and liver. Our bodies can also convert the betacarotene in orange fruits and vegetables and in leafy greens to vitamin A. To enhance the absorption of betacarotene, add some fat to the meal. For example, adding avocado or olive oil to a dish containing carrots or kale will help your child's body use the betacarotene more efficiently.
- **Vitamin D:** Although mainly derived from sunlight, vitamin D is also found in oily fish, liver, eggs and mushrooms. In winter it is likely your child will need a supplement, as we tend to cosy up inside during the shorter, colder days. Because vitamin D is fat soluble, the body is able to store it. Before supplementing, it can be worth talking to your doctor about a blood test to check your child's levels.
- **Butyric acid:** A naturally occurring fatty acid (found in butter), butyric acid helps to heal the gut wall, reduce inflammation and balance the immune system. Our friendly gut bacteria can produce butyric acid by fermenting certain fibres in the diet. So make sure your child's diet includes plenty of good-fibre foods: oats, flaxseeds, vegetables including leafy green vegetables, and grains such as quinoa, millet, buckwheat and brown rice.
- **Collagen and glucosamine:** Making your own bone broth (see page 190) provides both these important compounds, which can nourish the gut lining. Use the bone broth in homemade soups and stews, or as a warming drink just as it is.

There are also a few supplements that can be especially helpful for the restoration and repair of a leaky gut:

- **Colostrum:** Colostrum from grass-fed cows is an effective gut-healing supplement. It contains epithelial growth factor and a number of immunoglobulins, nucleotides and nutrients that lower inflammation and reduce any unwanted microbes. Colostrum powder is readily available, and is perfect for adding to all sorts of recipes – although it's not suitable for those with a dairy allergy.
- **Glutamine:** This amino acid acts as a major fuel for the cells of the intestinal lining. Offer it as a powdered supplement added to smoothies or stirred into yogurt or fruit purée.
- **N-Acetyl-D-glucosamine (NAG):** A naturally occurring amino sugar found in large concentrations in intestinal mucus (which is important for a healthy gut lining), NAG plays a key role supporting a healthy immune response. Found naturally in seafood, it is also available as a supplement – although you should avoid offering it to your child if he or she has a shellfish allergy.

Boosting your child's gut flora

Your child's gut is home to all sorts of different bacteria – including *Bacteroides*, *Enterobacteria*, *Bifidobacteria* and *Lactobacilli*, and there are many more – all of which, through their interactions with the immune system in our gut, help to promote oral tolerance (see page 42). They also help to maintain a healthy gut barrier (see page 64) and increase intestinal IgA (see page 56).

Children with allergies have been shown to have greater abundance of *Staphylococcus*, *Clostridium* and *Escherichia* bacteria species in their gut than non-allergic children, and significantly

Probiotic supplements

Probiotic supplements given to pregnant women and their babies have been shown to reduce the risk of the baby going on to develop common food allergies. In addition, they may even reverse certain reactions in children whose allergies have already developed. For example, in infants with an allergy to cow's milk, supplementation with *Lactobacillus rhamnosus* enabled tolerance to milk proteins, reversing the previous reaction. In older children with cow's milk allergy, supplementing *Lactobacillus rhamnosus* increased the body's production of IL-10, an anti-inflammatory cytokine, and alleviated allergic symptoms.

A word of warning: probiotics and histamine

If histamine appears to be a problem for your child, select probiotic supplements carefully. Histamine is a major component of the immune response and often associated with allergic symptoms. Certain microbes in our gut also have the ability to produce histamine. These microbes produce an enzyme called histidine decarboxylase, which converts the amino acid histidine present in various proteins into histamine. The more of these microbes your child has, and the more histidine he or she consumes, the higher the amount of histamine his or her body will produce in the gut. If your child is unable to get rid of that excess histamine effectively, the build up can trigger the same symptoms as those associated with allergies.

So what can you do? Keeping the gut flora healthy can help crowd out these bacteria and naturally help lower a child's histamine levels. This is particularly effective if you also take steps to help your child's body in its histamine detoxification (which may include offering enzymes to help break it down) and avoid eating high-histamine foods. Probiotic supplements can help, too, but some strains can actually produce histamine while others will reduce levels. Histamine-producing strains include *L. reuteri*, *L. casei* and *L. bulgaricus*, while those that help lower histamine include *L. rhamnosus*, *L. plantarum* and *Bifidobacteria*.

lower numbers of *Lactobacillus* and *Bifidobacteria*. Similarly, children with lower levels of various *Lactobacillus* species (*L. rhamnosus*, *L. casei*, *L. paracasei*) and *Bifidobacterium adolescentis* during their first two months of life were found to be at a higher risk of developing allergies to cow's milk, egg white, and "inhalant" irritants, such as pollen and dust mites. It appears, then, that the balance of your child's gut flora is crucial to establishing a healthy gut and reducing not only the symptoms of allergy, but perhaps even the incidence of allergy itself.

Fermented foods: Fermented foods (and probiotic supplements; see box, above) can help bring the gut flora and the immune system back into balance. Examples of fermented foods include sauerkraut, homemade pickles, kimchi, yogurt, kefir, kombucha, miso, natto and tempeh.

Gut-healthy fibre (prebiotics): Fibre found in certain vegetables (such as asparagus, garlic, Jerusalem artichokes, kale, leeks, onion, plantains, sweet potato, yams, leafy greens like broccoli and bitter greens like chicory and radicchio), beans and pulses, oats, flaxseed, and stewed apple (stewing helps break down pectin fibre making it more bio-available) help to feed friendly gut microbes. Known as prebiotics, gut bacteria ferment these fibres and produce short-chain fatty acids (SCFAs), such as butyrate (see page 62), acetate, and propionate, which regulate the immune system.

These foods are sometimes termed prebiotics, which just means they are rich in indigestible carbohydrates that reach the colon intact and selectively feed the many strains of beneficial bacteria there. Prebiotics are generally classified into three different types: non-starch polysaccharides (such as inulin and fructo-oligosaccharide), soluble fibre (including psyllium husk) and resistant starch. Each of these types of prebiotics feeds different species of gut bacteria, so think big and broad. Here are some ideas to get a wide range of prebiotics into your child's diet.

- Use onions and garlic in soups, casseroles and slow-cooked dishes. If your children will eat raw onions, add them to salads or slow cook and use to top homemade burgers or add to sauces and dips. You can also slow cook onions to sweeten them and add them to homemade breads and muffins.
- Use bananas, including less ripe ones, in smoothies or homemade banana bread and muffins.
- Sweet potatoes are incredibly versatile – they are great as wedges; mashed; grated into rosti; or spiralized to make noodles.
- Make up a batch of stewed apple as a healthy snack to have with natural yogurt or coconut yogurt.

- Use potato starch, inulin flour, green banana flour and chicory root powders in recipes for breads, cookies and crackers.
- Try adding salad greens, such as radicchio or chicory, to soups, salads and frittatas.
- Use canned beans in soups and casseroles, add them to salads, make them into burgers or mash them up in dips.

Polyphenols: Polyphenols are naturally occurring antioxidants found in many plants. Once they have broken down in the gut, they help proliferate friendly bacteria, while at the same time reducing potentially harmful microbes. Cramming as many of these foods into your child's diet as possible is an excellent way to improve gut health.

Polyphenol-rich foods

Many of the foods in the following list appear in the recipes in this book. But you'll see from the vast array of them that you can easily introduce them into a child's diet in many ways.

Apples • Blackberries • Blackcurrants • Blueberries • Broccoli • Cherries • Chestnuts • Flaxseeds • Globe artichokes • Grapes (red and black) • Hazelnuts • Nectarines • Olives (black and green) • Peaches • Pears • Pecans • Plums • Prunes • Tea (green and black) • Raspberries • Red onions • Spinach • Strawberries

Chapter 5

Tackling linked conditions

As if tackling food allergy itself weren't enough, it's very common for it to go hand in hand with a range of other childhood conditions. Although the focus of this book is food allergy, I want to highlight some of the closest links in order to give you a rounded view of what might be going on with your child's immune system. As so many things in life, a health condition rarely exists in isolation.

Eczema

Although eczema (also known as atopic dermatitis) affects people of any age, children seem to be especially vulnerable. In fact about three-quarters of sufferers develop the condition in the first year of their life. Children can also have a hard time refraining from scratching the itch, which of course makes things worse. Conventional eczema treatments usually involve anti-inflammatory skin creams that dampen the severity of the rash and itchiness, but do not actually address the cause.

Studies show that up to 40 percent of children with moderate to severe eczema have food allergies. In many cases, it is the food allergy that is a key cause of the eczema. Common culprits are eggs, cow's milk, wheat, soybeans and peanuts. Removing the food triggers (your child may need blood tests or to follow an elimination diet to establish which foods are the problem) and taking steps to address immune and digestive imbalances may improve things. In addition:

- Keep the skin dry and moisturized; allergens and microbes can easily enter the body through cracks in affected skin. Organic coconut oil (coconut is a fruit not a nut, so is often tolerated by those with tree-nut allergies), olive oil or refined shea nut butter (which appears not to pose any risk to those with peanut or tree-nut allergies) rubbed over your child's skin after a warm bath can help, especially if the bath itself is laced with Epsom salts, which contain skin-healing sulphur compounds. MSM (see page 56) sulphur creams may also help.
- Boost vitamin D through as much exposure to sunlight as is safe for your child, and increasing food sources, including cod liver oil, egg yolks, mushrooms, oily fish, and liver. Vitamin D helps to moderate levels of the bacteria *Staphylococcus aureus* on the surface of the skin – overpopulation is associated with skin flare ups.
- Add probiotics into your child's diet and in supplement form (see page 64), as certain strains – such as *L. rhamnosus* and *L. paracasei* – have been shown to improve eczema symptoms.
- Make sure your child's diet is rich in antioxidant vitamins and healthy fats. Vitamin A and beta carotene (in broccoli, butter, carrots, eggs, liver, spinach and sweet potato) and vitamin E (in avocado, nuts, olive oil, seeds and spinach) are known to be important vitamins for strengthening and maintaining the skin. Fish oils (omega-3 fatty acids in anchovies, herring, mackerel, salmon, sardines and so on) are anti-inflammatory and may help reduce eczema symptoms and flare ups.

Asthma

Many of the most common food allergy symptoms include sniffling, sneezing and excessive mucus formation. These can be linked to a variety of conditions of the airways such as asthma, rhinitis and sinusitis. Asthma often begins during childhood. It is primarily an allergic condition because allergens promote the release of histamine and leukotrienes – chemicals that lead to difficulty breathing, shortness of breath, coughing and wheezing, among other symptoms.

There are a number of potential underlying triggers for asthma – food allergies being one of them, as well as certain food additives such as sulphites (see page 26). Identifying allergens, strengthening the immune system and reducing symptoms can provide longer term relief. Take steps to replenish your child's gut flora and gut-barrier health, too (see page 63). In addition:

- Following a more Mediterranean style of eating (rich in plant-based foods such as fruits and vegetables, whole grains, legumes and nuts, and fish and a limited amount of red meat) has been shown to improve symptoms and lower the risk of asthma attack. Encourage your child to eat apples, too. Apples are rich in polyphenols and other compounds thought to protect against asthma symptoms.
- Boost vitamin D, which plays a crucial role in balancing the immune system and lowering the inflammatory reactions involved in asthma. Studies show that children (and adults) with asthma generally have lower levels of vitamin D in their system, and that pregnant women with higher levels of vitamin D had children with lower risks of wheezing and asthma compared with women with lower levels.

Key nutrients and their sources to help relieve asthma

If your child suffers from asthma, the following nutrients can help to support the health of the respiratory tract, balance the immune system and relieve symptoms.

- Vitamin C, for example found in citrus fruits, berries, red pepper, kiwi fruit and leafy greens.
- Vitamin D, for example found in egg yolks, oily fish, cod liver oil and liver.
- Vitamin E, for example found in almonds, sunflower seeds, sweet potato, avocado, spinach and wheat germ.
- Magnesium, for example found in leafy greens, pumpkin seeds, beans and lentils, brown rice, fish, almonds, dark chocolate and raw cacao powder.
- Selenium, for example found in Brazil nuts, sardines, beef, liver, turkey and chicken.
- Zinc, for example found in seafood, red meat, spinach, pumpkin seeds, cashew nuts, cocoa powder, beans and mushrooms.

- According to some studies, antioxidants (including vitamins C and E, flavonoids, selenium and zinc; see box above) can help reduce the bronchoconstriction associated with asthma. Magnesium can help improve lung function and relax the bronchial muscles leading to better asthma control.

- Try increasing the levels of anti-inflammatory nutrients in your child's diet. Omega-3 fatty acids, found in oily fish, flaxseed, chia seeds and walnuts, are particularly beneficial. Other natural anti-inflammatories include curcumin (see page 54), lycopene (found in tomatoes) and flavonoids (particularly quercetin, pine bark and *Boswellia serrata*). Another useful option is a supplement of butterbur. This is a perennial shrub used since ancient times as a healing plant. It has been shown to lower inflammatory compounds associated with asthma.

Hay fever (allergic rhinitis)

Hay fever affects about 20 percent of the UK population, and not just during the pollen season. If symptoms occur throughout the year, we call it perennial allergic rhinitis and it can be mistaken for a persistent cold. Various studies have demonstrated a link between allergic rhinitis and various IgE-mediated food reactions, including reactions to rice, citrus fruits, and banana.

Various studies show that using certain probiotics – particularly *Lactobabillus casei* – can decrease symptoms, reducing your child's need for medication. Other studies show that a mixed-strain probiotic, which includes *Bifidobacterium longum*, may help suppress inflammation and rebalance the immune response. Furthermore, nutrients that lower histamine can help relieve the symptoms of runny nose and excess mucus. Try a supplement of spirulina powder added to smoothies or stirred into soups and stewed fruit. Traditionally, stinging nettle has been used to treat allergic rhinitis, normally as an extract, but it is also available as a tea; or use the nettles in delicious soups (they lose their sting once cooked) just as you might kale or spinach, for example.

Hives (urticaria)

Food allergy is a recognized trigger for hives, along with certain metals and chemicals. In some children it's in fact an allergy to nickel – which occurs naturally in some foods and can leach into food from cookware – rather than food itself that causes the symptoms. Some research suggests that low levels of vitamin B12 and iron can also be a cause, and there are links with coeliac disease, so look out for gluten, too. You can treat hives naturally by avoiding the culprit foods and other triggers, and providing a diet rich with natural anti-inflammatories and antihistamines (see box, page 74).

Oral allergy syndrome

This is a type of food allergy classified by a cluster of allergic reactions in the mouth (symptoms are limited to the mouth, lips, tongue and throat) in response to eating certain (usually fresh) fruits, nuts and vegetables. It typically develops in hay-fever sufferers.

The condition is also referred to as "pollen-food-allergy" because a cross-reaction (see page 22) occurs between foods and inhaled allergens (typically pollen). Oral allergy syndrome is an IgE-mediated immune response (see p.ooo), so the body's immune system produces IgE antibodies against pollen that then bind to (or cross-react with) other structurally similar proteins found in botanically related plant foods. It can occur at any time of the year, but it is most obvious during the pollen season. For those with this condition, symptoms appear within minutes of eating the trigger foods. The most common reactive foods are apples, cherries, peaches, plums and nuts, such as hazelnuts and walnuts. Some children (and adults) also commonly have a latex allergy.

As this reactivity is IgE-mediated it may not be possible to completely switch it off, but it is possible to lower the level of reactivity with immune-modulating support, similar to the approaches outlined for asthma (see page 70). Improving digestive secretions (stomach acid and digestive enzymes) can also be helpful (see page 58).

What is histamine?

Histamine is an important chemical needed for the efficient functioning of many body systems, particularly the digestive system, the nervous system (including the brain), and the immune system (which releases histamine when fighting pathogens and allergens). The body needs certain enzymes to break down histamine, and in order to manufacture those enzymes we need to make sure we eat a diet rich in vitamins B complex and C, and minerals such as copper. If excess histamine appears to be a problem in your child's body, you need to reduce his or her consumption of histamine-forming or histamine-releasing foods, or of any foods that block the body's ability to manufacture the histamine enzymes. Alcohol and tea are the worst culprits when it comes to enzyme-blocking, so are less of an issue in a child's diet. Nonetheless, reducing processed meats, fermented foods and pickles, dried fruit (apricots, dates, figs, prunes, raisins), most citrus fruits, aged cheese (including goat's cheese), certain nuts (including cashews, peanuts and walnuts), certain vegetables (avocados, aubergine, spinach and tomatoes), smoked meats, and fish will all help. When we have too much histamine circulating in our bodies, we get the telltale symptoms of allergy – hives, itchiness, sneezing, runny nose and watery eyes and so on. Interestingly, some children might have a histamine intolerance rather than a true food allergy – it can be very difficult to identify the difference, and diagnosis will usually mean a laboratory test and/or an elimination diet, just as it would for food allergy. A diet rich in antihistamine foods (many herbs and spices, as well as apples, peaches, pomegranates, watercress and pea and bean sprouts are all good) can help to reduce symptoms.

Part Two

Getting down to business

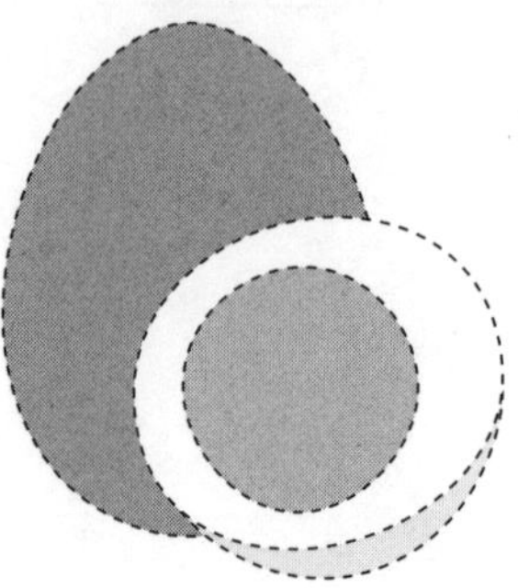

Understanding the nature of food allergy is just the beginning. Getting a diagnosis for your child is the first step on the road to managing and navigating food allergy in practical ways. This part of the book is about positive acceptance and positive action. It's about acknowledging the impact of the allergy and getting to grips with what it means for your child as the patient, you as his or her parent, and all of you as a family. In Part Two, we're going to look at embarking upon the food allergy journey with proactive confidence.

Whether your child received a diagnosis following an allergic reaction or was finally diagnosed after months of debilitating tummy problems, wheezing or skin rashes, the adjustment to living with a food allergy can be overwhelming. But, having an allergy is a whole-family experience – and I like to think of that as A Good Thing. It is something that you're going to learn about and conquer together.

Chapter 6

Talking and sharing

When your child is first diagnosed, it's perfectly normal to feel a whole host of emotions – from anxiety to fear to guilt. If your child has been diagnosed after a severe, life-threatening reaction, or you know this is a possibility, you may even be full of panic. But, this is no time to panic. Remember: this is the time for positive action to minimize the risks and even perhaps reduce the symptoms of allergy. This chapter is about dealing with the emotional rollercoaster of diagnosis in practical and accessible ways.

Listen and learn

First things first: your child will learn from you. However you feel inside, the best thing you can do for him or her is to take a positive, solution-based approach to what you know. Think about the language you use when you talk about the allergy – it's not about what you can't eat, but what you can; it's not a limited menu, but an opportunity to discover really exciting foods that we might never otherwise have tried; it's a culinary adventure we're going on together. Demonstrate that positivity in functional ways: select a few simple recipes in this book, cook and eat together, and gradually build up a range dishes that the whole family can enjoy.

Second of all, please don't blame yourself – the fact that your child has a food allergy is not your fault. And, anyway, you can't change what is – your goal now is to address any underlying imbalances in your child's immune system, create a culinary action plan, follow it and tackle the food reactions and symptoms head on.

Finally, find support. For yourself, for your child, and for anyone else in the family who might be confused about what it all means. There are online forums not only relating to food allergies in general but for specific reactions, and for coeliac disease, too. Make the process of discovery and learning something you do together. For example, you could ask everyone in the family to write down a question they have about the allergy and put it out to an online forum. Discuss the responses you get together – do you agree or disagree with what other people are saying? How do other people's experiences make you all feel?

Practically, support groups, national charities, local networks and your healthcare professionals will be able to help you to learn how to navigate your child's allergy safely and confidently. In this book alone you will learn what to look out for on food labels, and how to shop for and cook nourishing dishes for your child no matter what is off the menu.

Getting your facts right

The first step to feeling in control of the situation is to make sure you – as parents and carers – are clear about the type of reaction your child has and its implications. Any medical diagnosis can feel baffling for a child, even a teenager. *At the moment*, your age, life experience and remoteness from the condition itself mean that you are in the best position to gain a full understanding of what's happening in your child's body and to be able to reinforce and reassure as necessary. Sometimes being the person going through the diagnosis makes it harder to see the full picture of what that diagnosis does – and doesn't – mean.

Friends and family

There are practical reasons why you need to let other family members know about your child's food allergy – not least if any of them might ever have to cook for your child. Days out or sleepovers with grandparents and aunts and uncles need to be as safe as being at home. In addition, inherited allergies might be reflected elsewhere in your family – not only in your child's siblings, but in cousins, perhaps, too.

Apart from the practical reasons for sharing the diagnosis with your family, though, it's also really important to lean on others emotionally. When you're worried, call on your friends and family and ask for their support – to listen to you, to ask questions and to help you find the answers. Having someone outside the immediate situation can give you perspective and ideas that you might not think of yourself.

And don't feel rushed into leaving your child's meals in the hands of someone else – even someone you trust implicitly. Particularly when your child is very young, it can feel like a huge and overwhelming step to allow another person to look after your child and feed them. Do it at a pace that feels right for you and your child. Initially, that might mean trusting only your partner to cook for your child instead of you, then perhaps your parents, and eventually – when you're ready – trusted friends.

Ask yourself the following questions. If you can answer them, and you understand what your answers mean, you're already ahead of the game. If they reveal gaps in your understanding, that's entirely to be expected. The start of a food-reaction journey is a bombardment of tests, results and information. Make notes of the things you're uncertain about and arrange a time to see your child's doctor or dietician to really get to grips with what you're being told. You can do this with or without your child present – depending upon his or her age and level of understanding, and personality. Sometimes children get to grips with what's going on when their parents talk to them in terms they best understand; at other times children are more likely to take information on board if it comes from someone (anyone!) other than a parent. Make a judgement based on what's right for your family.

Ask yourself:

- Does your child have an IgE-mediated food allergy, a food sensitivity, a food intolerance or coeliac disease?
- Do you understand the underlying body functions and immune-system reactions that are causing the problem? Could you explain it to someone else? (It can be a good idea to try – often the questions that come back will give you a sense of how much you already understand, and anything you need some more information about.)
- Does your child have related atopic conditions, such as eczema or asthma, that you also need to manage? How are these physiologically related to your child's food reactions? (Ask yourself this to get a sense of how much you've been told about immune function.)
- Does your child have other digestive issues that you need to address? If so, what are they? What, if any, information has your medical team given you about how to address those issues?

"Why me?" Supporting and empowering your child

Even at a very young age, children can sense that certain foods may not be safe for them to eat. Once a child is diagnosed, it rarely takes a long time, even for toddlers, to become aware that they cannot eat the same foods as other children.

Supporting your child begins with being honest about their situation. Children are masters at sensing when they aren't being told the whole truth, and that's unsettling. Honesty makes a child feel safe. Be straightforward, practical and positive, and give your child an opportunity to ask you questions about his or her diagnosis and also let you know how he or she is feeling, too. Never dismiss a question or concern as "silly" or irrelevant. Children's minds work in ways that often seem random to grown-ups. Always validate their feelings and give appropriate answers to questions. If your son tells you he's scared his friends will make fun of him when he can't eat what they do at a party, tell him that it's okay to be worried, and offer him strategies for coping with his concerns, including giving him food options that he can eat. If your daughter is worried about saying no to foods at a friend's house, reassure her that very few people – even grown-ups – are comfortable saying no to others, but that it's really important that she learns to do so. Reassure her that if she's polite and honest, explaining her reason (that she has food reactions), grown-ups will respect that and you will be really proud of her. Give her some stock phrases to come out with. Allowing children to talk and ask questions empowers them to feel in control of their food reactions.

Explaining the allergy

There is no perfect way in which to convey the relative seriousness of an allergy, but trust that you know your child best: your instincts as a parent to provide information in the right way for your child are your best guide. Sharing information early on will help build trust. It also models acceptance of the diagnosis for your child.

Do, though, choose your words carefully. Children need to understand the implications of an allergy without becoming fearful. Depending on your child's age, here are some basics to cover, both in terms of explaining the allergy information and encouraging your child to act responsibly as he or she grows up.

Babies: 0–2 years

In this period, the responsibility for avoiding culprit foods belongs to you, and anyone else involved in your child's daily care. As your child's understanding and communication improves, start introducing the notion that not all foods are safe for them.

- Identify foods that are "safe" and "not safe". (At this stage, "not safe" should include borderline foods, too, so as not to complicate matters too much.) Cut out pictures from magazines or use play food to make up matching and identifying games.
- Use simple explanations, such as pointing to a picture of an egg and saying "Ow!" Use yes and no gestures (remember that even young babies can understand that a shake of the head means no and a nod means yes).
- Introduce the concept of "my milk", "Daddy's milk" and "[your child's name's] milk". Use brightly coloured stickers to indicate whose is whose.

- Be consistent: if you're using colours to identify good foods and bad foods, follow that through in everything you do – red for stop and green for go are obvious choices.

Preschoolers: 3–5 years

Because this is the age when most children start to stray from the 24/7 watchful eye of a parent, it's more important than ever to ensure that they have an independent understanding of what's safe and what's not for them to eat. Even if that understanding is rudimentary.

- Use child-friendly words and terms: "safe", "not safe", "sore tummy", "poorly skin" and so on.
- Use books to identify which foods your child needs to avoid, or cut pictures from magazines or use play food. Spend time (it need be only a few minutes at a time) sorting pictures into groups of "safe", "not safe" and "not sure". Learning which foods are in the "not sure" list is just as important as learning which ones are definitely in and definitely out. Make it a game, not a chore. And use colours – again, the traffic light system is a good one (red for not safe, green for safe and amber/yellow for not sure). You can draw or download picture outlines of foods, too, and encourage your child to colour them in the appropriate colour.
- Find websites with games and puzzles for children with allergies, and buy books and learn songs – there are lots of resources online, or make songs up to familiar nursery tunes.
- Use role play, both as a way to encourage your child to grow in confidence about asking about food, or saying no when offered foods he or she can't eat; and to learn to express what he or she feels when something is wrong. Teach phrases such

as "I can't eat pasta", "Cakes make me poorly" or "Milk makes my tummy sick." Remember that the notion of ingredients or components of food (gluten and even eggs) are hard for a child to understand – after all, to a three-year-old a cake looks like a cake, not an egg. Don't make too many leaps of logic. (If you're making egg-free cakes at home, teach phrases such as "I can only eat mummy's cakes.")

- Use simple language for explaining symptoms and ask your child to use those words back to you: "My mouth feels hot", "My arms feel itchy", "My mouth feels sticky."
- Identify key staff at nursery or playgroup whom your child can go to if he or she feels poorly when you're not there. Encourage those people to ask your child questions relating to how he or she feels: "How's your tummy today?" "Do you feel itchy?" and so on. Build trust between them, perhaps playing the allergy-teaching games that you and your child play at home. Nursery staff will have undergone allergy training – it is useful to spend separate time going through their procedures and, in broad terms, reassure your child that they know what steps to take if he or she feels poorly.

Young school-age children: 6–12 years

Sometimes having more understanding about what's going on in the world creates more anxiety, and feelings of being out of control. So, at this age, supporting your child through their diagnosis and the first part of their journey is all about empowerment.

Young school-age children are old enough to be far more aware of their "differences" than babies and toddlers. With this age group, be open, honest and even adult in your explanations. Don't use complicated language or words, but start to explain the science behind what's happening. Use books with pictures of the body and anatomy in them. Look up key words online or in an encyclopaedia or dictionaries: immunity, allergy, gluten and so on. Remember that knowledge is power – for your child as well as for you.

Developing independence is so important during this phase in a child's life, and even more so when diagnosed with a lifelong allergy that your child will need to learn to manage him- or herself. Teach your child about his or her medical kit, if you have one. Demonstrate how to use the autoinjector and explain what it does and why it's important. Find a bag to carry it in that your child is proud to hold – it needs to be an extension of them, and go everywhere, so find something he or she loves.

Make personalized safety cards together with important emergency information on them: what the allergy is, what the reactions might be, what to do in an emergency, and who to call. These are especially important if your child is not yet ready to verbalize – perhaps through shyness or embarrassment – what he or she can and can't eat. Little "business cards" with name and headshot, and lists of can eats and can't eats are really useful for handing out in restaurants or giving to friends and family. Encourage your child to decorate the cards with drawings and stickers (if age appropriate), or design them online together.

If your child needs to wear a medical alert bracelet, encourage him or her to remember to put it on themselves: make it part of the morning routine – have breakfast, brush your teeth, collect your bracelet and your medical kit.

Cooking with children, including encouraging them to make their own packed lunches, is a practical way in which you can empower your child to feel in control of his or her allergy. The more children learn about food and understand how to use and cook with it, the more interested and knowledgeable they are. Not only do they learn about food, but studies show that cooking encourages more adventurous eating and that children become more aware of how to prepare foods safely and (in the case of kids with allergies) avoid cross-contamination. Putting together meal plans (see pages 171–7) with your children also helps them to feel part of the family mealtime process, rather than different from it.

Expose your child to different social situations – eating out, parties, family gatherings, barbecues and so on – so that he or she learns through experience to assess risk and make appropriate selections. Choose places to eat out together and encourage your child to order his or her own food, and to inspect it and to ask the serving staff questions about it, if need be. Use role play to prepare

Make things routine

Children respond to patterns in their day. And when something is routine, it stops being something different or peculiar, and is just part of daily life. While it's important that your child realizes he or she must be careful, it's also important to normalize things as much as possible. Be consistent in your instructions and repetitious. Tell your child:

- Always carry your auto-injector.
- Always check labels.
- Eat only foods that have a clear list of ingredients that you can check.
- Don't eat anything you're uncertain about.
- Never swap foods or try anything from someone else's plate.

your child for these social occasions if it would help – after all, it can be hard to query an adult when you're not even a teenager yet.

Teenage life

You may think that the worst years are when your children are very young. However, arguably it is the teenage years that cause parents most concern. In adolescence, teens face peer pressure – and all the while their brains are developing and their hormones surging. Adding food allergies to greater independence ratchets up the risk-taking potential: not all teens willingly speak up about culprit foods. At best this is because they want to fit in and fear being different, at worst it's a way to rebel. However, it's worth highlighting that teenagers with food allergies are often more responsible and more empathetic towards others, and – given the opportunity – tuned in to the notion of self-care. Many teenagers demonstrate an impressive ability to take responsibility for themselves and be accountable for their behaviour, when their parents give them the freedom to do so. For many parents, though, this is the hardest challenge of all: letting go. As difficult as it may be, we have to recognize that it's ultimately our teens' responsibility to begin to take care of themselves.

Parenting a teen requires a significant shift in how you offer care and support. A young child needs protection; a teen needs independence and the opportunity to take responsibility for themselves. To complicate matters, simply talking to teens about risks won't necessarily change behaviour. Teens need room to make their own decisions. So, rather than trying to tell a teen what to do, start by simply providing information – lists of can-eats and can't-eats and a reminder of the early warning signs of reaction. Give your teen his or her medical kit (with instructions). Talk about the importance of carrying it around at all times (this is

Reducing risk at teen parties

We already know that teenagers are risk-takers (they are wired that way – it's an important developmental stage), but a teenager with an allergy still needs to understand that some risks are not worth taking. Social situations are among the hardest things for teenagers to navigate at the best of times, and even more so when there are certain allergy rules controlling the fun. Here are a few top tips to help your teen reduce risk when the party season kicks in:

- Eat before the party – if you aren't hungry, you don't need to risk food you're not sure about.
- Drink only from your own cup and eat only from your own plate.
- Find an ally – make sure at least one friend at the party is aware of the allergy, supportive of its implications, and able to react if something goes wrong.
- Learn about alcohol: beer contains gluten and many cocktails and liqueurs contain dairy or eggs.
- Never put the auto-injector in the pocket of a jacket or coat – carry it at all times. Get a neat little pouch that will attach to a belt. Where you go, the epi-pen goes.
- Be aware of the dangers of kissing: a teen with a severe peanut allergy, for example, could react to the peanut residue on the lips or in the mouth of the person at the other end of the kiss.

an important reminder that comes with increasing independence throughout your child's life). Where and how does he or she intend to carry it around, and do they remember how to use it in an emergency? It's important that they always feel confident about using their epi-pen. Try to find incentives to motivate him or her to act on what they know about their allergy, and make sure he or she knows that your door is always open for questions and support whenever they need it, but never put pressure on them to talk.

Many teenagers feel awkward or shy discussing their allergies. Help your teen plan ahead for social situations. This could include collecting menus from local restaurants and calling to speak with staff ahead of time (encourage your teen to make the call). Come up with some set spiels for ordering food: "I just wanted to let you know I have a number of severe allergies, so my food cannot contain or come into contact with any of these items. Can you let me know on the menu which items are safe please, or can you make changes to certain dishes to accommodate my allergies?"

Peer support

Having a supportive friendship group is particularly important for teenagers. Look online together to find local support groups for teens with allergies or coeliac disease. Finding like-minded peers can be a particularly good confidence boost and may even provide a social network. Give your teen access to social media, too. There are growing numbers of blogs and Facebook groups specifically for teens with allergies. Remember that social media is the place where young people readily exchange information and experiences. Ultimately, engaging and educating peers, and learning from other allergic teens, helps to create a stronger, safer environment for your own teen, and with it, over time, greater social acceptance.

School life

Just as it is important to speak to children about their allergies, it's really important to have good communication with your child's school staff. When your child starts a new school and at the beginning of each school year, make an appointment with the head teacher, the class teacher and the school nurse to talk about what your child is allergic to and what to do if he or she has an allergic reaction.

Don't be afraid to ask questions at these meetings: they provide your opportunity to speak to those involved in your child's care and to hear about their experiences in looking after children with allergies. You need to make sure they are fully confident to deal with your child's needs, and that they will be able to read the signs and symptoms that might present in your child. Take with you any information you have from your child's allergy appointments. For severe IgE-mediated food reactions, you should have a "food allergy emergency care plan", which sets out what to do if your child has an allergic reaction. Give a copy of this to the school staff. If your child needs an auto-injector, the school nurse and trained staff should have two on the school premises. Make sure you involve your child in these school meetings, too, so they feel included and understand what to do and whom to go to if problems arise at school.

School meals

School mealtimes often cause anxiety throughout the chain of responsibility, from child to parent to the school staff. My first piece of advice is to speak to the school caterers yourself to ensure

IgE-mediated food allergy: what school must know

If your child has a risk of anaphylaxis, spell out to their school how to recognize an anaphylactic reaction and when and how to administer adrenaline or other medication. Provide your child with a medical alert bracelet if you are worried. Make sure your child's teachers know to:

- Ensure there are two auto-injectors with your child and that they know how to use them.
- Administer a second shot, if symptoms don't improve within 10 minutes of the first.
- Always take your child to hospital, even if the auto-injector has relieved symptoms and your child seems better.

the school canteen is aware of your child's allergies and the importance of providing safe options for him or her. Ask to see the kitchens and talk about cross-contamination. Make sure you're convinced that the hygiene is rigorous and that the importance of maintaining it absolutely clear.

If you're worried, most schools allow children (whether they have allergies or not) the option of bringing a packed lunch rather than eating a school meal. I've included lots of packed-lunch ideas in the book, all of them nutritious and interesting (no more limp sandwiches!). Similarly, send your child in each day with an allergy-free snack to minimize risks.

Other children's food

One very difficult thing to police is what other children bring to school as snacks or in packed lunches. Don't rely on nut-free policies at any school. While caterers can provide assurance that meals do not contain nuts, it is impossible to police every packed lunch brought in for hidden allergens. Ask the school to raise awareness among other families and in the meantime educate and empower your child to have the confidence to tell others what they are allergic to and to discourage any food sharing.

If your child has cookery lessons at school, speak to the teachers about alternative ingredients and a separate area for preparing and cooking foods to avoid the risk of contamination.

School occasions

In many schools it is common practice to share a birthday cake or sweets on special occasions. There may be other times, such as festivals or international celebration days, when new foods are shared in class.

When you speak to your child's class teacher at the start of the term, explain that you'd like warning of any occasions that the class will celebrate in order that you can provide alternative foods for your child to enjoy at the same time as everyone else, so that he or she can join in. The potential for a child to feel isolated and different while everyone else is chomping away on something is immense. It is often useful to arrange with the school a "safe food box". You provide the box and a few safe, culprit-free treats for your child. That way, if there's a birthday that you didn't know about, your child's teacher can find something from the box that your child can eat with his or her classmates.

Parties, play dates and sleepovers

No child should feel awkward or embarrassed about going to a party and not being able to eat the food. One thing I would say: there will always be a handful of children at a party who won't eat what's put in front of them, simply because of personal likes and dislikes – a child with allergies almost certainly needn't feel alone.

Take control. If your child is invited to a party, let the host know when you accept the invitation about his or her allergies and tell them you'll drop off a special party tea when you arrive. Ask what sorts of things their party tea will serve up and offer to bring similar allergy-free food to take the pressure off the host. Some parents will even be happy and confident to make something special for your child themselves – especially if it's as simple as swapping in gluten-free bread or pasta, for example. But many will be grateful not to take the risk. Good hosts will never be offended if an allergic child refuses food. Reinforce the idea of saying no politely before your child goes to the party, so that he or she feels confident when there.

If your child is staying overnight at a friend's house, offer to provide plenty of provisions to cover breakfast, as well as other meals and snacks. Use a cool bag, if you need. Keep foods wrapped or sealed within the containers and label them clearly. Remember to pack drinks, if relevant, too. Before you leave your child, make sure the host knows what to do if your child has a reaction and leave labelled medications just in case. Ask if he or she would like a list of culprit foods, and make sure you provide your mobile phone number. This is not only essential in case of emergency, but if the host is concerned about a certain product he or she is serving up, they can take a photo of the food label and send it to you to check yourself.

Chapter 7

At home

Caring for a child who has been diagnosed with a food allergy is a whole household – even lifestyle – experience. From the moment that you know there are certain foods that are now out of bounds for one (or more) of your children, and even while you're still processing the news, you'll need to get organized. First, you'll need to know how to shop so that you know what you're looking for, then you'll need to make sure that your kitchen cupboards are not only full to brimming with can-eats, but properly sorted so that it's clear who can eat what. Wherever you are and whatever you and your children are doing, you'll need to be well-prepared enough that what goes onto your child's plate is not only a *suitable* meal for him or her, but delicious and nutritious, too.

This section will give you all the top tips and techniques, as well as nutritional know-how and delicious substitutes you need to ensure that at home, eating out, and going on holiday (among myriad other scenarios) is yummy, healthy and fun for everyone. It will take you through the key bits of information you need to start living a way of life that is suited to having a child with food allergies, but that doesn't feel in the least bit burdensome (for anyone). We'll look at:

- Deciding how to approach an allergy diagnosis at home – is allergy-free food going to be for one, or for all?

- Sorting out your kitchen and how to organize your cupboards to ensure that the right foods are in the right places and labelled in the right way.
- Deconstructing your utensil drawer to ensure that you minimize the risk of cross-contamination.
- Preparing food safely, serving it safely and having everyone at the table together eating safely.
- Shopping economically and healthily with allergies in mind.
- What to expect from restaurants – and how to ensure kitchen and serving staff understand your family's needs.
- Pre-empting requirements during holidays abroad, and what you'll need with you in case something goes wrong.
- All the major allergens and their perfect substitutes, not just like for like on a plate, but in terms of being able to conjure up goodies such as cakes and biscuits for a child who can't eat wheat or egg, for example.
- Top tips, advice and examples on how to ensure the removal of any food doesn't result in nutritionally depleted meals – after all, children need to grow and thrive and it's our job as parents to make sure that that's exactly what they do, no matter what health limitations there are on their diet.

Deciding on your approach

For many families, the simplest, clearest and most failsafe approach to ensuring that home is not a place that exposes children with allergies to foods they can't eat is to remove the culprit foods completely. That is, everyone eats in the same, allergen-free way. For example, if one child is diagnosed coeliac, the whole family switches to a gluten-free diet; if a child is diagnosed with a nut allergy, your home becomes a nut-free zone.

There are lots of benefits to choosing this approach. For example:

- Bread, flour, pasta (or milk, ice cream and custard) and so on in the cupboards are safe for everyone, so there's no risk of confusion or error, and no need to label packets individually.
- There's no cooking different meals for different people.
- A child with allergies has one less environment in which he or she feels singled out in some way.
- The risks of cross-contamination are removed, or at least significantly reduced.

It sounds a no-brainer, but it's often not really that simple. A free-from diet is not necessarily right for everyone in the family, and in some cases (particularly where siblings are involved) can become a source of resentment. In addition, while it is absolutely possible to keep the cost of free-from foods down, there is still no denying that a loaf of store-bought regular bread is cheaper than even homemade gluten-free bread. (But, then, if you're making it, why not make it for all?) There are nutritional considerations when it comes to some free-from diets. Undeniably, it takes a bit more initial effort to ensure nutritional balance in, say, a dairy-free diet than it does in one where calcium-rich milk and yogurt are on the menu.

Only you can decide what's right for your family. Consider:

- First and foremost, the severity of the allergy – if you have a child whose first reaction will be anaphylaxis, it may make it easier and less stressful if the whole family goes allergen-food free. If, on the other hand, you can minimize cross-contamination, establish rules that everyone will follow and reactions are mild, perhaps having a dual-diet household isn't going to be a problem.

- The family dynamic – do you have other children who may struggle with avoiding certain foods? Will your allergic child feel left out if you don't all adopt the same diet? Remember that when you're eating out, your other children may not need to avoid everything that is out of bounds at home, so they need not be completely gluten or dairy free.
- How much time do you have to make separate meals?
- How adventurous or open-minded are your children's palates – bear in mind that while it's perfectly possible to provide a fully rounded diet using replacement foods, sometimes that means eating a broader range of foods than some children will immediately find acceptable – if they have a choice.
- How organized are you as a family? Will everyone understand the cross-contamination rules and be able to stick to (or remember) what is suitable for whom if you have a mixture of foods in the cupboards?
- If you start out with mixed cupboards, could you switch to a free-from diet by stealth? For example, most good-quality gluten-free pasta tastes very similar to regular pasta and the chances are no one will even notice.

The truth is that we are so much better at understanding how to substitute deliciously and nutritiously than we were even five years ago, so over time it's likely that you can create a free-from household without anyone feeling that they are missing out or compromising. While your instincts might tell you to rid your house of all allergen foods with immediate effect, if your child's reactions allow, perhaps the softer approach will have longer-lasting benefits for everyone. I have found that, among my clients at least, naturally free-from becomes the norm for the whole family, over time.

Remember: It's not just foods you need to be mindful of. Common food allergens can also be present in certain medications, supplements, hair-care products, creams and beauty products (including make-up), and even play-dough.

Storing food safely

When you first think about rearranging your kitchen cupboards to accommodate your children's allergies, it may feel utterly daunting. However, think of it as a new beginning. A sort of kitchen catharsis, if you will.

Start by emptying everything. Then, with a cloth and bowl of warm, soapy water or eco-friendly kitchen cleaner, wipe over, under and inside every cupboard until your kitchen is spotless and crumb free. Allocate which cupboards or shelves are to be for which foods. If you're keeping some cupboards for non-allergen-free foods, perhaps you might put signs up on the outsides, or label individual shelves. It might not be the latest trend in interior design, but even as a temporary measure it will help everyone get used to the idea that there are clearly determined places for certain foods. If you have young children, this is a great way to get them involved – ask them to draw you pictures to put on the front of a cupboard that is especially "theirs", for example.

Then, start going through everything you've emptied. If you're going household allergen free, throw away (or allocate to a food bank, if you can) anything that's on the banned list (along with throwing away anything that's been lurking so long it's out of date). Wipe down the outsides of jars and other packaging of everything you're keeping with a soapy cloth and, if you're allocating kitchen space to allergen-free/allergen foods, put every jar, can, packet into its appropriate cupboard so that you store all free-from foods away from regular foods. Make sure, where necessary, allergen-free foods are in labelled and sealed jars or sealed plastic containers. (Don't forget to check manufacturer labels as you put things back – in particular, spices and condiments may contain allergens that aren't immediately obvious.) I promise, once you've finished and everything has a spotless storage space, you'll feel like you've conquered the world.

The fridge

Once you've tackled the cupboards, tackle the fridge. Keep free-from foods, such as dairy-free milk and spreads, in sealed containers and on a separate shelf in the fridge, away from allergens, such as butter, cheese and so on. Use the same procedure for frozen and chilled foods – keep them in a separate area and seal them in separate, clearly labelled containers or bags.

Cooking safely

If you've decided that following two dietary plans is suitable for your family, you need to get rigorous when you cook, because in some cases cross-contamination (when traces of food are left on preparation and cooking equipment) can be enough to cause a reaction, or (in the case of coeliac disease) damage the delicate villi that line the gut (see page 31). But, don't worry, there are lots of tips and techniques to help you to establish and remember the rules, and before long cooking safely will feel like second nature.

Preparing food

- Always prepare the free-from foods first, ideally up to the point that they are ready for cooking.
- Do make sure you keep the utensils and cutlery you're using for the allergy-free recipe separate, and make sure they have been thoroughly washed – ideally in a dishwasher, if you have one, or in hot, soapy water – to ensure that no lingering traces of potential allergens remain. If you find it easier, you could have two sets of utensils and two sets of cutlery – one dedicated to free-from prepping and eating, and one for everything else.
- Use differently coloured chopping boards for free-from foods, and even use a particular colour cloth to wipe down surfaces.
- Wipe down surfaces before you begin preparing food – use hot, soapy water or an eco-friendly cleaner – and wash your own hands thoroughly.
- Use separate baking trays, dishes, pans and so on for free-from foods.
- When it comes to washing up, wash pans, utensils, cutlery and crockery in hot soapy water or on the hot cycle in your dishwasher.

Cooking food

- Use separate shelves in the oven for free-from and culprit foods, placing free-from foods above anything else (this ensures that if there's any dripping or spilling during cooking, there's no chance of contamination from above). If you have a double-oven, you could even dedicate one of them specifically to free-from cooking.
- When you're baking or grilling, use baking parchment to cover oven trays and racks before you cook – you can throw these away after cooking and replace with fresh next time.

Storing the auto-injector

If your child's reactions are severe and he or she carries an auto-injector, make sure everyone in the family knows where it's kept and train everyone who is old enough how to use it. Also make sure that everyone knows to put it back in the same place. Make it clear that this is not a toy, but an important medicine that can save a life. If you leave your children with babysitters, ensure they know where the medicine is, when and how to use it.

- Use a separate toaster for gluten-free breads, or use toaster bags in shared toasters and sandwich machines.
- Use separate saucepans, where necessary, and stir using separate spoons or other utensils.

Sitting down to eat

It seems so obvious to have to store food and cook separately if someone in your family has an allergy. However, what may seem less obvious is ensuring that during mealtimes, as a family you minimize the risks of cross-contamination. Many of the following tips are just good table hygiene anyway, so no one need feel singled out for special or alternative treatment, but you'll know that not only are you teaching your children impeccable table manners, you're also protecting the members of your family with allergies.

- Make sure everyone washes their hands before they sit down to eat and as soon as they leave the table.

- Create a family seating plan that ensures that children who are eating different foods are positioned opposite each other, or away from each other, especially if they are particularly messy or likely to try to taste foods from each other's plates.
- When dips, condiments, spreads, or help-yourself foods are on the table, you'll need to make sure any serving cutlery doesn't become contaminated with culprit foods. Decant sauces and condiments into little bowls with spoons of separate colours, or encourage children to choose and allow you to serve them, so that you can add a dollop or a squeeze while taking care to ensure you don't touch allergen foods as you serve. Alternatively, allocate your allergic child his or her own tub of, say, spread or jam, label it securely and ensure that no one else helps themselves to it.

Chapter 8

At a restaurant

While cooking and eating at home are fully within your control, there are lots of situations where children need to be able to eat out. We cover school, playdates and parties in Chapter 6, but here I want to talk about restaurants. European and UK law require eateries across all European countries to let customers know which foods on their menu contain any of the 14 primary allergens (see page 123). However, there is no regulation as to how this information might be conveyed, which can make eating out incredibly stressful, particularly in the early days of diagnosis, when you're just getting used to the kinds of questions you need to ask on behalf of your child (and your child is getting used to the idea of having to ask these questions for him- or herself).

Some restaurants, for example, will train their waiting staff to convey information about allergen foods on their menu directly to their customers in response to queries; others might add labels, highlights or symbols to the menu; in takeaway restaurants, labelling might be on the counter, on signage or in fridges next to food itself. Many restaurants will have special allergy-free menus to make choosing appropriate dishes as straightforward as possible – you just need to know to ask for one. Over the following pages, I'll give my top tips on how to keep eating out the fun experience it should be.

Choosing a venue

Some restaurants – and cuisines – may be better suited than others for catering for people with allergies. For example, restaurants that cook everything to order, from scratch rather than buying in prepared sauces and other menu items are usually good choices. Think boutique café rather than fast-food chain. Thai cuisine is great for gluten free, but not so good for those who can't eat shellfish or eggs. Lots of South American food is also naturally gluten free.

Preparing ahead

I love the fact that these days most restaurants post their menu on a website or Facebook page for my family to check out before we head to dinner. Look ahead before you book and share the menu with your child, so they are confident there's something they'll like and have an idea of what to order. It is also a good idea to warn the restaurant when you book that you have a child who has allergies with you. Given notice, lots of eateries will happily make sure they have something suitable and delicious available.

Before you leave home, consider taking surface wipes with you. You can minimize the risks of cross-contamination in restaurants and cafés by wiping down tables (and high chairs or baby seats, if relevant) before you sit down.

Arriving and ordering

You are your child's greatest teacher and arriving at a restaurant and checking that his or her needs are clear is one of the most important things you can teach – in time, he or she will have to do the same for themselves. When you arrive at the restaurant, tell the front-of-house staff that your child has allergies and state very clearly what they are. Repeat the information to waiting staff when they bring the menus, and again when they take the order.

When you order, ask questions if you need to double check ingredients. For example, ask whether sauces are thickened with wheat flour, or whether fried foods are dusted in flour before frying. If your child is dairy free, ask whether butter is used as an emulsifier in sauces or to coat vegetables before they come to the table. Have eggs been used to bind burgers or as a glaze on meats or breads? Ask about cooking oils – many restaurants will use nut oils for frying, or in dressings or condiments; and ask whether curries, for example, use fish sauce, which often contains shellfish. (Again, checking the menu before you arrive can help you think about the kinds of questions you might need to ask. Don't be afraid to take a crib sheet if it helps.) If you're worried, keep your child's order simple – go for grilled fish or chicken with a selection of vegetables and a plain baked potato (specify no butter, if dairy is a problem) or plain rice, for example.

When your order arrives, double check with the staff that they're confident your requests for allergen-free ingredients have been followed, and check to make sure there aren't any sauces or extras that might have been added inadvertently and be problematic.

Excuse me, my child is...

Here are some key questions to ask staff when eating out with children with specific dietary requirements. Even if neither of these allergens is relevant for you, the diet-specific questions will give you a good sense of the sorts of things you need to ask for in your child's particular situation.

Dairy free

- Does the sauce, gravy or soup have added butter, cream, milk or yogurt. Have the croutons been fried or coated in butter?
- Will the soup be topped with a swirl of yogurt, creme fraiche or cream?
- What oil does the chef use for roasting and frying? Does the chef use a combination of oil and butter?
- Do any marinades contain dairy products?
- Are vegetables tossed in butter before serving?
- Are potatoes mashed with butter, cream or milk?
- Are the baked potatoes served with melted butter or does butter come separately?
- Are there any dairy products in the salad dressings?
- Is served bread dairy free?

Gluten free

- Are wheat flours used to thicken gravies and sauces, or in marinades?
- Does the chef use gluten-free stock cubes?

- Are meat or fish tossed in flour before roasting or frying? (Generally, watch out for floured, breaded, battered or crumbled dishes.)
- Can the restaurant supply tamari gluten-free soy sauce instead of regular soy sauce?
- What toppings are there on soups and salads? (Watch out for crumble mixes, added couscous or croutons)
- Are gluten-free foods cooked separately from non-gluten-free foods? In particular, are pizzas cooked separately?
- Do sausages contain gluten breadcrumbs? Similarly, stuffings, patties and burgers?

Chapter 9

Going abroad

With different cuisines come different cultural attitudes to foods, different "standard" ingredients, and different levels of understanding and rigour about food allergies and reaction prevention. I've been to some countries where an appreciation of the difficulties of food allergy is significantly greater than it is at home; and I've been to others where it feels like I'm having to explain everything as if food allergy were the most unusual ailment in the world. In general, though, worldwide understanding of food allergy is rapidly increasing, as experts estimate that more than 250 million people worldwide are sufferers, more of them children than adults. Nonetheless, even where understanding is improving, labelling standards vary wildly, so my advice is: always be prepared.

It's all in the planning

Take time to research the country you want to visit and find out about any common allergens that might appear without a second thought in that country's cuisine. For example, Thai food often contains fish sauce (often made with shellfish) or shellfish powder; Malaysian and Indonesian food often contains peanuts (think chicken satay); Mexican, Italian and French foods are often heavy on cheese or gluten. It doesn't mean you shouldn't visit those countries, it just means you will need to be especially vigilant when asking about food before it's served to your child. Find out about the healthcare in the country you intend to visit and how easy it will be to access emergency medicine. It is important to have travel insurance that will cover allergic reactions, including anaphylaxis, and related medical conditions.

Most allergy and coeliac associations have special travel advice packs and dietary alert cards you can carry with you when travelling.

Accommodation

Think about whether or not self-catering might be better for you as a family. But, if you want the full hotel experience, before you leave speak to your travel company or the accommodation company itself about provision for special dietary requirements. If you hit a problem with understanding before you even leave, consider whether or not this is the right location for your family. How easy you find it to gain reassurance before you leave is a good indication of how easy you'll find it once you arrive.

In-flight safety

If you're flying, check the airline's policy about allergens in the aeroplane meals. (Many airlines avoid having nuts in anything they offer, for example.) And some airlines operate a "buffer zone" (usually three rows behind and in front) around passengers with severe allergies, asking passengers around your child not to eat anything containing the particular allergen. If you're very worried, you can ask to pre-board to wipe down seats, trays and arm rests to remove any food residue. It's also worth asking if the airline trains its staff in the treatment of anaphylaxis and carries auto-injectors on board (although, of course, you should always carry your own supplies of necessary medications in your hand luggage;

see box opposite). I recommend that you always carry with you a recent doctor's letter confirming your child's allergy. Although you won't necessarily need it, some airlines and airline staff will ask to see it before accommodating special requests, such as making an announcement to ask passengers to refrain from eating nuts, peanuts or other allergens during the flight.

However, remember that no matter what moves an airline makes to reduce the risks associated with allergies, none will guarantee you a completely allergen-free flight (for the simple fact that it's impossible to control everything the general public consumes). Do your research, choose an airline that seems the most accommodating and always be prepared to treat any symptoms or reactions during your flight.

Food for the journey

If you are at all worried about the reliability of an airline to provide allergy-free food, take food with you. Although liquids (including yogurts) won't be allowed through check-in, most items you'd put in a packed lunch (see page 168) will be fine. Some airlines will warm your food for you in their in-flight microwaves, but don't count on it. Cold salads, wraps and sandwiches, made at home in the environment you know is safe can be just as delicious. Use cool bags (bear in mind ice packs are filled with liquid, so won't be allowed on a flight), partly to maintain the temperature of what you pack, but also to seal the food away, keeping it safe from cross-contamination. And don't forget allergen-free snacks, too. Always take more than you need – travel can be fraught with delays. Even if you're travelling by car, don't rely on motorway service stations to provide allergen-free foods. Have things covered for yourself.

Hand-luggage rules

Always carry your child's allergy medicine and auto-injectors with you in your hand luggage. Remember to carry antihistamines or other medication in containers under 100ml, although larger bottles are allowed for medical purposes. Make sure you have a letter from your doctor and a current prescription list with you in case of any disputes at check in.

Inform the staff – everywhere

When travelling, it is worth telling the staff about your child's allergies when you book, when you check in, and when on board. Repeat all that information when you arrive at your accommodation and remember that staff will change over the course of a day, and probably over the course of a week. Never be afraid of repeating yourself! If you're putting your child in holiday club as part of a package deal, remember to let all those who will be caring for him and her know, every day if you need to. Don't assume that information is passed from a travel agent to on-site staff, or from one set of staff to another – be prepared to share everything anew. Finally, don't forget to check that staff are appropriately trained in dealing with any allergic reaction and have the right medical kit to ensure your child is always in safe hands.

Chapter 10

Building a nourishing free-from diet

We all want the best for our children. Not only do we long for them to be happy and fulfilled in life, equipped with a range of social and life skills and with the confidence to reach their full potential, we also want them to be well-nourished so that they can live a life that is as healthy as it can be.

From the moment they're born, we're told that what we feed our children has a profound effect on their overall health and well-being. Energy levels, brain function, behaviour and intelligence are just some of the many and varied aspects of our children's well-being that are affected by what we feed them. It's for this reason that following a diagnosis of an allergy, so many of the parents I see begin the free-from journey in a state of despair.

Arguably, it's even more important that children with allergies get adequate amounts of vital nutrients that are so crucial to the health of their immune system, their developmental process overall, and in shaping their health long term than those who are born allergy free.

I know from experience that making changes to a child's diet – particularly in a way that you've perhaps never had to think about in your own life before – can feel overwhelming. There are certain nutrients that you may need to focus on, and other tweaks you may need to make to ensure that everything you feed your child is nutrient dense to make up for any deficit that comes from not being able to eat certain other foods.

To begin, I've listed some top suggestions for all children who need to follow a free-from diet, regardless of the specific allergy. Take each change one at a time, where possible introducing changes gradually. Always persevere if your child is finding one particular change hard to accept – some foods will take several attempts before children will accept them (and I've found this is as much the case for allergy-free children as it is for those with allergies – some challenges are just plain parenting!).

Focus on the balance

The balance of food groups on your child's plate is the first place to start. Aim to cover half the plate with a rainbow of colourful vegetables – they can be raw or cooked. Packed with phytonutrients, vegetables can be really crucial to feeding beneficial gut bacteria and keeping the gut healthy. Appropriate (that is allergen-appropriate) lean protein (eggs, meat, fish, chicken, beans and pulses, soy, nuts and seeds) should cover a quarter of the plate, and the remaining quarter should include some starches. Good examples are starchy vegetables (carrot, parsnip, swede, sweet potato, yam or cassava) and whole grains (rice, quinoa, millet, buckwheat, oats and so on).

Hold the sugar

We all need to be aware of the levels of sugar we consume. Sugars are found naturally in foods such as fruit, vegetables and grains, or as lactose in milk products, but sugar is also commonly hidden in refined versions in many everyday foods and contributes to obesity, weight gain, blood-sugar imbalances and dental decay. For those with allergies it's worth knowing that many shop-bought free-from foods ramp up flavour by increasing sugar content. Sucrose (table sugar), syrups and high-fructose corn syrup are common culprits.

The best way to keep sugar levels low in the foods you feed your children is to cook from scratch. For recipes that need sugar (such as cakes and biscuits), switch to sweeteners that release energy slowly into the blood stream (low glycemic index sugars), such as xylitol, stevia and erythritol. Note that honey, maple syrup and black strap molasses although natural are not necessarily healthy, so try to use them in moderation. Avoid fruit juices and sugary drinks and instead opt for water, or milk or dairy-free milk alternatives as drinks for your children.

Add in foods that support gut health

We learned in Chapter 4 that supporting a healthy gut is one very important way in which to try to balance your child's immune system to minimize the body's response to allergens wherever possible. Fermented foods are hugely beneficial for helping the gut to populate with the good bacteria that is so important for gut health. Try to include kefir, kimchi, kombucha, miso, natto, raw pickles, sauerkraut, tempeh and yogurt in as many family meals as possible. While some may seem a little exotic, there is such a variety that you are likely to find many options you will all enjoy.

Similarly, include sources of prebiotics. Cooked pulses (beans, lentils and peas), green bananas, plantains and potato starch, as well as asparagus, chicory, dandelion greens, garlic, Jerusalem artichokes, jicama, leafy greens, leeks and onions are all good choices.

Your children will need plenty of fibre to support gut health, too. Avoid refined "white" grains – switching to wholegrain options will provide more fibre and nutrients for your child.

Recipes to support gut health

- Homemade soups (pages 216–219), such as Chicken Noodle Soup (page 218)
- Apple Sauerkraut (page 197)
- Berry Kefir Shake (page 200)
- Falafel Bites with Salsa and Minted Dip (page 222)
- Slow-cooked Beef Chilli (page 234) with Cornbread (page 236)
- Chicken Schnitzel with Coleslaw (page 247)
- Harissa Traybake Vegetables and Chickpeas with Herby Yogurt (page 266)
- Tropical Parfait (page 272)
- Easy Chocolate Mousse (page 273)
- Berry Apple Crumble (page 275)

Keep up the healthy fats

No healthy-weight child – whether suffering from food sensitivities or not – needs to be put on a low-fat diet. The right types of fat are vital nutrients for children to develop a healthy brain, good eyesight, and a healthy nervous system. In addition, the healthy fats, particularly the essential omega-3 fatty acids and monounsaturated fats (found in avocado, olives and nuts) reduce inflammation and help modulate the immune response and support gut health – all of which are especially important for children with allergies. As long as your child isn't allergic to fish, boost healthy omega-3 fats through a diet that includes oily fish and shellfish two or three times each week. If you need to avoid shellfish, try vegan options, which include chia and flaxseeds (delicious stirred into porridge or as a part of a crumble topping) and walnuts, daily.

As well as good fats themselves being an important part of a healthy diet, certain nutrients, such as vitamins A, D, E and K, are fat soluble and found in fatty foods. Deficiencies, particularly in vitamins A and D (found in organ meats and cod liver oil, in particular), can affect gut health and immune tolerance to antigens.

Avoid pro-inflammatory fats, which include hydrogenated or trans-fats commonly found in processed foods, ready meals and deep-fried foods. Unless they are a culprit food, use butter, nut and seed butters or coconut oil as healthy spreads. Replace vegetable oils with olive oil or cold-pressed organic rapeseed oil.

Recipes packed with healthy fats

- Vegan Buckwheat Seed Bread (page 188)
- Carrot Cake Granola (page 201)
- Breakfast Seed Bars (page 208)
- Salmon Kedgeree (page 213)
- Mexican Taco Chicken Salad (page 229)
- Chowder Fish Pie (page 253)
- Creamy Prawn Tikka Masala (page 257)
- Sweet Potato Salmon Fish Cakes (page 259)
- Tropical Parfait (page 272)
- Buckwheat Seed Crackers (page 280)
- Creamy Guacamole (page 283)
- Lemon Chia Shortbread (page 287)

Don't skimp on protein

All children need protein for the development of their muscles, tissues and enzyme scaffolding – in fact protein itself is like the scaffolding of the entire body. For children with allergies it's especially important for a healthy gut barrier (see page 000) and immune system. Choose high-quality meat protein from organic, grass fed, free-range sources, and the same goes for eggs. Choose wild rather than farmed fish and seafood. Plant sources of protein include beans, pulses, soy, nuts, seeds, superfoods (such as spirulina) and pseudo grains (such as teff, quinoa and amaranth).

Recipes packed with protein

- Breakfast Bean Burritos (page 209)
- Breakfast Sweet Potato Chorizo Hash (page 210)
- Baked Beans On Waffles (page 211)
- Salmon Kedgeree (page 213)
- Chicken Noodle Soup (page 218)
- Falafel Bites with Salsa and Minted Dip (page 221)
- Homemade Pasties (page 224)
- Pineapple & Pork Salad (page 225)
- Mexican Taco Chicken Salad (page 229)
- Slow Cooked Beef Chilli (page 234)
- Chow Mein (page 237)
- Fruity Lamb Tagine (page 239)
- Pesto Meatball Pasta Bake (page 241)
- Pulled Jerk Pork (page 243)
- Barbecue Traybake Chicken (page 245)
- Chicken Schnitzel with Coleslaw (page 247)
- Moroccan One-pot Chicken with Rice (page 249)
- Courgette/Zucchini Noodle Carbonara (page 251)

- Chowder Fish Pie (page 253)
- Fish Bites with Homemade Tomato Ketchup (page 255)
- Creamy Prawn Tikka Masala (page 257)
- Sweet Potato Salmon Fish Cakes (page 259)
- Smoky Bean Burgers (page 264)
- Spicy Chickpeas (page 284)

Spices and herbs provide not only flavour (enabling you to avoid salt and sugar), but an array of anti-inflammatory plant compounds that help to soothe an overactive immune system.

Chapter 11

Shopping and cooking

Even once you've sorted out your kitchen and got the patter right for when you're eating out of the house, the day-to-day practicalities of living with a child with food allergies are ongoing. There are lots of ways in which you can start to form a rhythm to your week so that the things you have to think about when you're shopping, and preparing meals themselves, come to feel perfectly normal and natural for the whole family.

Be inspired

Never underestimate the resources around you – whether they are the meal plans and recipes in this book, or the ideas and tips you'll find on allergy-related social media groups and allergy websites and forums. Make use of your doctor, dietician or nutritionist or allergy clinic for additional resources, too. Talk to the assistants in your local health food shop, and find local allergy or coeliac groups to meet with others in comparable situations and to swap stories and advice.

Plan your meals

Planning your weekly meals is more important for families with children with allergies than it is for anyone else. Planning what you're cooking and eating every day will help you to avoid risks and temptations while you're out shopping and ensure you have everything you need at the end of the shop. You'll save money, not only by being less susceptible to temptation as you wander around the store, but because cooking free-from meals from scratch, rather than relying on potentially expensive shop-bought free-from products, is generally cheaper.

When you're out shopping...

Read the food labels

Once you are aware of your child's food allergies, becoming savvy with reading food labels needs to become second nature. In the UK and Europe, food manufacturers must, by law, clearly highlight in bold, underline, large font, or colour the 14 major allergens (see box, opposite), if they appear in the ingredients of any particular product.

Sometimes front-of-pack statements make claims for the food as "free from" certain allergens (for example, foods may be labelled "gluten free" and so on). Although helpful, these statements are entirely voluntary, so I advise that you always check the ingredients list, too. A vegan symbol means that it contains no animal products – including dairy, eggs, fish and shellfish – but always check the label for other allergens, too. Never stop checking labels and don't make assumptions. Remember that product specifications often change, so keep vigilant. Check the websites of registered allergy charities and organizations, too. Many will ping up alerts when

The 14 major allergens

The following are the 14 major allergens identified on UK and European packaging, by law.

Celery (including celeriac) • Cereals containing gluten (wheat, barley, rye, oats, spelt, kamut) • Crustacea (such as crabs, crayfish, lobster and prawns) • Egg • Fish • Lupin • Milk (including lactose) • Molluscs (such as cockles, mussels and oysters) • Mustard • Peanuts • Sesame • Soy beans • Sulphur dioxide and sulphites • Tree nuts (almond, Brazil nut, cashew, hazelnut, pecan, pistachio, macadamia nut, walnut)

manufacturers make changes to their products, helping to keep you informed.

It is also worth mentioning that just because a product is labelled as suitable for those with particular food allergies, it does not mean it is *healthy* for your chid. Many free-from products are often highly refined and nutrient poor, and can upset a child's blood-sugar levels. While prepared foods, such as free-from breads, can be useful, I would encourage you to make things from scratch as often as you can – that way you can take full control of not only the allergy-free aspects of your child's diet, but his or her nutritional intake, too.

Fresh is often free-from

Shopping for food-sensitive children does not have to be complicated or expensive. The key is to focus on whole, unprocessed real foods and to shop in the free-from product aisle only when you really have to. Focus on fresh fruit and vegetables with lean proteins and some healthy fats – with this in mind, you'll have a naturally free-from diet packed with nutrients but without the expense. (In some countries, including at the time of writing in the UK, if your child has been diagnosed with coeliac disease, a doctor can prescribe a certain amount of free-from products every month.)

For more unusual ingredients, make use of health food stores or online retailers. Be mindful of risks at delicatessens. While they may sell high-quality fresh produce, there is a risk of cross-contamination if assistants are carving and wrapping up individual orders. Check that the store has a policy of using separate boards, serving spoons and knives when serving (and that staff are following it). Pre-packing in plastic is slowly losing favour, but pre-packed foods will reduce the risk of cross-contamination in the case of allergies. To remain environmentally conscious, look for foods that are packaged in cardboard rather than plastic.

"May contain"

Food manufacturers commonly use the term "may contain" to cover themselves if there is a risk that the food has been contaminated with an allergen during the production process. Whether or not to include such a statement is voluntary and unregulated, so there is no way to know what the chances of contamination are. Only you can decide what risks are worth taking based on the severity of your child's allergy.

Shopping for your dairy-free child

If your child reacts to animal milks, he or she will need to avoid all dairy, including lactose-free dairy products. This is because the reaction is to milk protein, not to milk sugar. Look out for labels that highlight milk or cow's milk – some may also highlight butter, cream and yogurt – and avoid those products. Remember that milk from goat, sheep and buffalo may also be problematic for a child who is allergic to dairy, because these milks contain similar proteins to those in cow's milk. Ingredients such as whey, casein, caseinate, lactalbumin and lactose also indicate that the food contains dairy. If the product is labelled vegan, you know it will be dairy free.

Use the following tables to establish the main foods you'll need to look out for on food labelling, and then to identify suitable substitutions.

Dairy foods to avoid	Foods to treat with caution
• Butter • Buttermilk • Cheese, including cream cheese, mascarpone and cottage cheese • Cream, ice cream and crème fraîche • Custard (unless dairy free) • Lactose-free dairy products • Milk powder • Rice pudding, semolina, tapioca puddings • Whey protein powders • White sauce and béchamel sauce • Yogurt and fromage frais	• Batter products (including pancakes, Yorkshire puddings and tempura) • Breakfast cereals • Chocolate • Dressings • Flavoured snacks (including popcorn and crisps) • Fudge, toffee and caramel • Malted drinks and hot-chocolate • Margarines • Pastries, buns, cakes and so on • Sausages • Soups and sauces (including pesto)

Substituting milk products

Look for plant-based milk products that have been fortified with calcium, vitamin D and vitamin B12.

Children under four-and-a-half years old are not advised to have rice drinks as a replacement for cow's milk. Note that the nutritional quality of plant-based milks varies considerably. Use the information in the box below to help you choose the alternative that's most suitable for your child.

I need to substitute...	Try...
Milk (see also box, previous page)	• Almond milk and other nut milks (such as cashew, hazelnut) • Apple juice or fruit purée for flavour or binding in baking • Coconut milk and milk powder • Hemp milk • Oat milk • Rice milk • Soy Milk • Tiger nut milk (chufa)
Cream	• Coconut cream • Dairy-free custard powder • Nut creams • Silken tofu or blended firm tofu • Soy cream
Kefir	Coconut kefir
Yogurt or ice cream	• Coconut, soy or nut-milk ice creams • Coconut or nut yogurt (see pages 192–4) • Soy yogurt

I need to substitute...	Try...
Cheese	Vegan cheese (usually soya-based or made using nuts)
Butter	• For baking: Dairy-free spreads (such as those based on olive oil) and coconut oil; sometimes nut or seed butters • For spreading: Nut or seed butters or tahini; dips such as hummus or guacamole; or a drizzle of olive oil

Dairy-free nutrition

Milk is a useful source of protein, calcium, iodine, some B-vitamins, and a little vitamin D. The body needs all these nutrients, and while protein and B vitamins are readily available from other food sources (and non-food in the case of vitamin D, which we manufacture from our exposure to sunlight), it takes a little more effort to find iodine and calcium in sufficient quantities.

Finding iodine: Found primarily in fish, sea vegetables and dairy products, iodine plays a crucial role in brain health, development and metabolism. White fish actually contains more iodine than oily fish. Try adding sea-vegetable flakes into soups or stews, or sea-vegetable seasonings to scrambled eggs.

Finding calcium: Calcium is crucial for bone health so finding calcium-rich alternatives to milk for a dairy-free child is important. The recommended daily intake for children for calcium is between 350mg and 550mg, depending on age (the higher amount being for older children and teenagers). As a measure, one 200ml glass of cow's milk contains about 240mg of calcium; 30g of cheese

The best nutritional substitutes for dairy milk

The following are common substitutes for cow's milk and are useful to have in your armoury of dairy alternatives. However, not all milk substitutes are created equal. Think about what your child needs for his or her diet and choose an alternative that supplies the best nutritional content possible.

- **Almond milk and other nut milks:** Slightly higher in fat and protein than rice milks. Available fortified with B-vitamins, vitamin D and calcium. Not suitable for nut-free diets.
- **Coconut milk:** Canned full-fat coconut milk is high in calories and fat and not fortified. Natural source of manganese, magnesium, copper, potassium and lauric acid (a type of fatty acid that can help to support immune function). Carton coconut milk often is lower in fat and usually fortified with B vitamins, vitamin D and calcium.
- **Oat milk:** High in fibre. Not normally suitable for children on gluten-free diets.
- **Rice milk:** Low in fat and calories, watery tasting, low in protein. Available fortified with vitamin D and calcium. Not suitable as the main drink for toddlers.
- **Soy milk:** High in protein; often fortified with B vitamins, vitamin D and calcium. Rich-tasting so good for sauces and dressings.

- **Tiger nut milk (chufa):** Good source of healthy monounsaturated fats, vitamin E, calcium, fibre, iron, magnesium and phosphorous. Check labels and avoid products sweetened with sugar.

contains 220mg of calcium and 120ml of yogurt contains about 200mg of calcium.

Many dairy-free milks are now fortified with calcium (and vitamin D), helping to meet daily needs. Focus also on offering foods that are not only good sources of calcium in themselves, but good sources of calcium that your child's body will readily absorb. For example, while leafy greens are often rich in calcium, some of them are also high in oxalates, compounds that bind to calcium and reduce its absorption by the body. High-oxalate vegetables include spinach, beetroot greens and chard. Instead, offer kale, mustard greens, turnip greens and broccoli, which are low in oxalates. Use the following table to help you ensure your dairy-free child is getting enough calcium in his or her diet.

Dairy alternative	Calcium in mg
Sardines with bones (½ can)	258
Calcium-enriched milk alternative (200ml/7fl oz/ scant 1 cup)	240
Tofu (60g/2½oz)	200

Dairy alternative	Calcium in mg
Calcium-fortified instant hot oat cereal (15g/½oz/1 tablespoon)	200
Chia seeds (2 tbsp)	177
Calcium-fortified soy yogurt (125ml/4fl oz)	150
Sesame seeds (2 tbsp)	140
Tahini (2 tbsp)	128
Dried figs (60g/2½oz/½ cup)	120
Almond nut butter (2 tbsp)	111
Almonds (30g/1oz/¼ cup)	94
Kale, cooked (65g/2½oz/½ cup)	90
Pak choy/bok choy, cooked (75g/3oz/½ cup)	79
Orange (1 medium)	75
White bread (1 slice)	65
Kidney beans, cooked (75g/3oz/½ cup)	58
Hempseeds (2 tbsp)	57
Sweet potato, cooked (100g/4oz/½ cup)	45
Broccoli, cooked (75g/3oz/½ cup)	43
Chickpeas/garbanzo beans, cooked (75g/3oz/½ cup)	40
Black beans, cooked (75g/3oz/½ cup)	23
Lentils, cooked (40g/1½oz/½ cup)	19

Shopping for your egg-free child

A reaction to egg could mean that your child is allergic to proteins in the egg white, the yolk, or both. Because it's the make-up of the egg itself that's usually the problem, dieticians will generally advise that those allergic to eggs steer clear of all eggs, whatever the source. That means that your child should probably avoid eating not just chicken eggs, but duck, goose and quail eggs, for example, too.

Remember that egg is often used in products to bind, thicken or flavour them, or to provide additional protein. On labels, egg is often given other names: yolk, egg white, albumin, globulin, lecithin E322, ovomucoid, ovovitellin, livetin are all ingredients to look out for (and under UK and EU law must be highlighted in some way).

Egg foods to avoid	Foods to treat with caution
Eggs in all forms – cooked (poached, omelette, frittata, scrambled, boiled, fried and so on) and raw	• All baked goods – cakes, biscuits, pastry goods (including tarts and quiches) and muffins, for example • Batter (pancakes, Yorkshire puddings and so on) and battered or breaded foods (fish fingers and so on) • Breads, and sweet breads, such as brioche and glazed rolls • Custards, mousses • Egg pasta and noodles • Meringues • Royal icing, marzipan • Sauces, such as tartar, bearnaise, hollandaise and mayonnaise • Sausages, burgers and meatballs • Sorbets and ice creams

Substituting egg products

Avoiding eggs themselves (that is, as a boiled egg or scrambled egg and so on) is not such a difficult thing (for scramble, you could substitute with tofu). However, eggs are used in so many ways in all types of cooking – to thicken sauces, bind together other ingredients, in dressings, desserts and batters, or to help breadcrumbs to stick to breaded fish and meat, for example. My clients are often most daunted by the notion of trying to bake without eggs – after all, we use eggs in baking to help with leavening and as a binding agent, and to glaze buns and bread. However, there are alternatives, both commercially and using natural ingredients. Use the following table to help you substitute egg in all manner of cooking situations.

I need a substitute for eggs in...	**Try...**
Baking	Per egg, any of the following: • 1 tbsp agar flakes soaked in 2 tbsp hot water to dissolve • 60g/2¼oz apple purée • ½ banana, mashed • 1 tbsp chia seeds soaked in 3 tbsp water for 10 minutes before using • 2 tbsp chickpea flour in 3 tbsp water • 4 tbsp drained liquid from a can of chickpeas (known as aquafaba) • 1 tbsp ground flaxseed soaked in 3 tbsp water for 10 minutes before using • 60g/2¼oz/generous ¼ cup Greek yogurt, coconut yogurt or soy yogurt • 2 tbsp potato flour, arrowroot or cornflour

I need a substitute for eggs in…	Try…
Baking (cont.)	• 50g/¾oz/¼ cup prepared dairy-free custard • 1 tbsp pysllium husks soaked in 3 tbsp water for 10 minutes before using • 60g/2¼oz pumpkin purée • 60g/2¼oz silken tofu, blended • 1 tbsp soy flour in 3 tbsp water • 60g/2¼oz mashed or puréed cooked sweet potato or butternut squash
Dressings and dips	• Kefir or coconut kefir • Silken tofu • Soaked and blended nuts, particularly cashew nuts and macadamia nuts • Yogurt or dairy-free yogurt
Glazing	• Honey • Liquid gelatine • Maple syrup • Milk or dairy-free milk
Desserts	• Commercial custard powder, yogurt or dairy-free yogurt, whipped cream or coconut cream • As a setting agent: agar flakes or gelatine to set desserts, soaked and blended cashew nuts with coconut oil
Thickening	Cornflour, potato flour or arrowroot

I need a substitute for eggs in...	Try...
Binding	• For breadcrumbs: Coat moist chicken or fish in fine breadcrumbs or dip first in a little milk before rolling in the crumbs • For burgers, sausages or fish cakes: simply omit • For stuffings (per egg): 1 tbsp ground almonds, breadcrumbs or oats
Pastry	20g butter or dairy-free spread (or a little extra xanthum gum in gluten-free pastry)

Egg-free nutrition

Eggs are a useful source of protein (about 6–7g of protein per egg), so remember to give your child sufficient protein-rich alternatives at each meal; they are also a good source of vitamins A, B complex, D and E, as well as calcium, iron and phosphorous. For your child's brain health, eggs provide choline, which is a precursor to the memory neurotransmitter acetylcholine. Other choline-rich foods include organ meats, such as liver; certain oily fish, such as salmon, sardines and mackerel; and beef, turkey and chickpeas.

Shopping for your nut-free child (peanuts and tree nuts)

Peanuts aren't actually nuts – they're part of the legume family and classed as groundnuts (and may appear on labels as groundnuts, or groundnut oil). Tree nuts include Brazil nuts, hazelnuts, pistachios, cashews, pecans, walnuts, macadamia nuts, and almonds. Most nuts have the potential to cross react with one another (see page 22) and possibly with peanuts, too. Be mindful that children with a nut allergy may also react if they eat coconut-containing products or nutmeg, too (although links are rare). As peanuts are part of the legume family, occasionally you may find cross reactions with beans and pulses and even carob and lupin.

Nut and peanut foods to avoid	Foods to treat with caution
• Nuts and peanuts in all forms • Nut spreads and butters • Nut oils • Nut-based granola and breakfast cereals • Satay sauces	• Baked goods, including cakes, biscuits, savoury and sweet pastries, desserts • Curries • Dressings • Fried foods • Gluten-free products • Nougat, marzipan, praline • Stuffing mixes • Sweets and chocolate products

Substituting nut and peanut products

The best alternative to nuts and peanuts (and their products) is seeds (and their products). If your child can tolerate coconut, this is available in many forms and makes a brilliant alternative in baking. Nutritionally, seeds (and their products) will provide much of the goodness you can find in nuts.

I need a substitute for...	Try...
Whole or chopped nuts	• For baking and crumbles: Pine nuts, seeds, and coconut • For curries: as above
Nut butters (including peanut butter)	• Flavoured coconut oil • Seed butters • Tahini (sesame seed paste)

I need a substitute for...	Try...
Nut oils	• For Asian dishes: Sesame oil • In dips and dressings: Mixture of olive oil and sesame oil
Toppings or coatings	• Breadcrumbs • Buckwheat flakes • Crushed crisps, popcorn, rice cakes or corn crackers • Desiccated or flaked coconut • Ground-up seeds • Millet • Mixed seeds • Oats • Pine nuts • Polenta • Quinoa

Shopping for your wheat- and gluten-free child

Grains such as wheat, barley, rye, spelt and kamut all contain gluten. Furthermore, because of the ways in which foods are packaged and processed, oats are often cross-contaminated with gluten, so it's important to choose gluten-free oats, too. If your child's allergy is to wheat, rather than gluten, he or she should be able to tolerate barley and rye. All the recipes in this book are gluten-free, but do check ingredient labels as some less obvious products may contain gluten. For example, not all baking powders are gluten-free.

Manufacturers are required to highlight any gluten-containing grains in their products on the food label – look out for ingredients containing wheat, barley or rye. Products labelled "gluten free" must contain less than 20 parts gluten per million; "low gluten" labels mean that there is no more than 100 parts gluten per million but are rarely used in practice.

Gluten-containing foods to avoid	Foods to check carefully
• Barley • Bulgur wheat • Couscous • Farina • Kamut • Marmite • Matzo • Oats (often contaminated with gluten) • Rye • Semolina • Spelt • Triticale • Wheat • Wheat germ	• Biscuits, cakes, crackers, breads, pasta and so on • Breaded and battered foods, such as fish fingers, goujons, breaded chicken, meatballs, falafels • Canned beans in sauce, and canned soups • Cereal bars and breakfast cereals • Flavoured rice mixes • Frozen fries • Instant hot drinks • Ketchup and other condiments • Malt vinegar • Malted drinks • Marinades • Meats, such as ham, sausages, burgers and salami • Oats (unless certified gluten free) • Pastries • Quorn products • Roasted and coated nuts, seeds and crisps • Seitan • Soy sauce, teriyaki sauce • Stock cubes, gravy

You may see the statement "No gluten-containing ingredients" (NGCI) in shops and on menus. From February 2018, this statement is allowed only in relation to lists of products in shops and dishes on menus. Even though the items in the list are not gluten-containing foods, the shop or restaurant is not guaranteeing that they are gluten-free. Note that until February 2018, manufacturers could use NGCI on product labels – that's no longer the case in England.

Substituting gluten-containing foods

With so many gluten-free grains, pseudo grains, and starches, as well as prepared gluten-free flours available, the opportunity to substitute gluten-containing foods for your child is vast. I might even go as far as to say it's liberating!

I need a substitute for...	Try...
Wheat flour	• Almond flour • Amaranth flour • Banana flour • Bean flours • Buckwheat flour • Chestnut flour • Coconut flour • Gluten-free flour mixes (see page 182) • Gram (chickpea) flour • Maize meal / corn meal and cornflour • Millet flour • Peanut flour • Potato flour • Quinoa flour • Nut and seed flours • Rice flour • Sorghum flour

I need a substitute for...	Try...
Wheat flour (cont.)	• Soy flour • Tapioca flour • Teff flour
Grains and starches	• Amaranth • Buckwheat • Cauliflower or parsnip "rice" • Gluten-free oats • Millet • Quinoa • Rice (white, black and red) • Sweet potato and potato • Wild rice • Yams, cassava, yacon
Pasta	• Gluten-free pastas and noodles • Kelp noodles • Konjac noodles • Spaghetti squash • Spiralized carrot and courgette
Breads, crackers and snacks	• Bean and chickpea snacks (see page 284) • Buckwheat crackers and crispbreads • Dehydrated sliced fruits and vegetables • Flaxseed crackers, seed crackers (see page 280) • Gluten-free breads, rolls, pitta breads, wraps (see pages 184–9) • Gluten-free bread mixes (see page 182) • Gluten-free oat cakes • Homemade cornbread (see page 236) • Kale crisps • Paleo breads and muffins • Plain crisps or sweet potato and vegetable crisps (see page 282) • Plain popcorn • Raw crackers, corn crackers, rice cakes

I need a substitute for...	Try...
Thickeners	• Arrowroot • Cornflour • Mashed potato or sweet potato • Potato flour • Rice flour • Sago • Tapioca flour • To thicken soups and stews: cooked rice, quinoa or other grains, sweet potato, or potato
Breakfast cereals	• For homemade granola or muesli (see page 200): rice, millet, buckwheat, gluten-free oats, quinoa, puffed rice, puffed corn • For porridge (see page 206): millet, quinoa, buckwheat, rice and amaranth
Batters	• Gluten-free flour blend (see page 182) • Gram flour • Potato flour mixed with cornflour

Making gluten-free flour mixes

In wheat-flour baking, gluten helps bind ingredients together, trapping in air to create elasticity in dough and helping breads and cakes to keep a light texture and structure. In order to achieve these effects in gluten-free baking, you'll need different types of flour, different techniques and different baking times.

Gluten-free flours vary in their characteristics – from their protein content to their taste, density and texture. Some are higher in protein and heavier than wheat flours, but often more nutritious. Used on their own in baking, they can create a dense texture, so it's often best to combine them with lighter, starchier flours.

Different proportions better suit different cooking purposes. Some gluten-free flour mixes use 70 percent wholegrain flours and 30 percent starchy flours; others use a little more starch, which can be better for making pastry, for example. Here's a list of some of the most popular wholegrain gluten-free flours suitable for combining into your own gluten-free flour mixes (see also pages 186 and 236). (Once made up, gluten-free mixes will last for between three and six months in an airtight container.)

- **Almond flour:** Particularly high in monounsaturated fats, vitamin E, magnesium and potassium, almond flour is good for heart health – and makes delicious, dense cakes.
- **Amaranth flour:** A staple in the Aztec and Incan diets, amaranth is a protein-rich flour that provides plenty of the amino acid lysine, which can be low in vegetarian and vegan diets; good source of iron and fibre. Its higher starch content means it helps with binding.
- **Brown rice flour:** This is a useful light flour that is richer in fibre than regular white rice flour; a good source of B-vitamins and manganese; combines well with higher protein flours, such as sorghum, quinoa, teff and amaranth.
- **Buckwheat flour:** With its nutty, rich flavour, this flour is delicious in cakes, pancakes and breads; a good source of protein and fibre and rich in phytonutrients, including rutin, known for its antioxidant properties. I like using it with chestnut flour in cakes and muffins.
- **Chestnut flour:** Milled from dried chestnuts, this is a sweet and nutty flour that is quite starchy, so good for moist cakes and puddings.

- **Coconut flour:** High in lauric acid, a healthy saturated fat that is essential for immune health, healthy skin and good thyroid function. Because coconut flour comes from the meat of dried coconut, it's a good source of protein and fibre (which makes it good for gut health, too).
- **Millet flour:** This flour has almost the same protein content as wheat, and for that reason makes a good addition in bread mixes, but does have a strong nutty flavour. You'll need to combine it with starches, such as arrowroot or tapioca.
- **Nut flours (general):** Rich in monounsaturated fats, vitamin E, fibre, magnesium and potassium, nut flours provide protein in cakes and breads. You can even make your own: use a processor to grind up the nuts until you have fine crumbs.
- **Polenta:** Yellow in hue, polenta gives baked goods colour and moisture and, used like a high-protein flour, is delicious in cakes and muffins.
- **Quinoa flour:** A good addition in breads and pastry, quinoa is incredibly nutritious with 60 percent more protein than wheat, and provides a good source of the minerals iron, zinc, copper and calcium.
- **Sorghum flour:** A delicious option for breads and cakes, sorghum flour has a nutty, sweet flavour; its fine texture means it works well in cakes; high in antioxidants and fibre rich.
- **Soy flour:** High in protein, soy flour is a good addition to bread mixes to create more moisture and texture.
- **Teff flour:** Known for its high protein content, teff is also packed with potassium, calcium, iron and fibre. It has a lovely rich flavour, but can be dense, so combine it with lighter, starchy flours such as tapioca or potato flour.

Using gums

Not all gluten-free baking requires a gum, but it will help bind mixtures together, especially in pastries (see our shortcrust pastry recipe on page 183 and brioche bread recipe on page 186, for example). Popular options are xanthum or guar gum, but you can also use ground flaxseed, chia seeds or pysllium husks, or ground pectin powder. In some recipes you can use eggs, yogurt or milk to help bind, or some fat such as coconut oil or butter.

Gluten-free starches

- **Arrowroot:** I like using arrowroot as a binding starch in cakes, pastry and breads. It is also a great way to lighten breads.
- **Cornflour:** Made from very finely ground corn, cornflour is well known for its ability to thicken sauces, but I use it in pastry and breads, too.
- **Gram (chickpea) flour:** high in protein which can help mixtures to bind and is commonly used as an egg substitute. I sometimes use this in breads to help with binding as well as boosting the protein content.
- **Potato starch:** Made from peeled potatoes and very fine, potato starch helps provide a light but moist texture in baked goods. It's very starchy, so a little goes a long way.
- **Tapioca flour:** This starch has a sweet flavour and adds a silky texture to baked goods.

Gluten-free nutrition

For any child diagnosed with coeliac disease, a gluten-free diet for life is essential. However, by the time of diagnosis, children with coeliac disease often already have significant nutritional deficiencies, because the gluten they have been eating has been damaging the delicate lining of their gut (see page 000) and affecting nutrient absorption. One study found that 67 percent of patients with overt coeliac disease and 31 percent of those with a silent or subclinical case had malnutrition at the time of diagnosis. Common nutritional deficiencies in children and adults at the time of diagnosis include iron, calcium, B-vitamins and vitamin D. This makes it especially important to know how to boost your child's nutritional intake while also going gluten free. Remember, of course, that being gluten free in itself, especially if you rely on ready-made gluten-free products, will likely lower your child's intake of fibre and increase saturated fat, salt and sugar.

So, my first tip is one I've given before, but it's worth reiterating: base your child's diet on natural and unprocessed gluten-free foods, cooking from scratch whenever you can, rather than relying on processed free-from products. Then, take special care to include:

- **Fibre:** Gluten-free products are often more refined and lack essential soluble fibre, which many of us (children and adults alike) eat too little of anyway. Fibre is essential to support a healthy gut microbiome, and a healthy digestive tract. Good sources of fibre include green leafy vegetables, beans, pulses, flaxseeds, chia seeds, gluten-free whole grains (quinoa, millet, wholegrain rice, buckwheat) and skin-on sweet potato, as well as nuts and seeds.

Coeliac disease and your child's bones

Bone disorders are more common in children with coeliac disease. This is partly linked to an increase in malabsorption (failure to fully absorb nutrients from the gastrointestinal tract) of bone-building nutrients and increased inflammatory response in the body. Damage to the small intestine can particularly affect the absorption of vitamin D and calcium, but may also affect the assimilation of other fat-soluble nutrients involved in bone health, such as vitamin K.

For healthy bones your child needs a wide range of nutrients including vitamin C, vitamin D, vitamin K, magnesium, boron, silicon, zinc and protein, as well, of course, as calcium. You can provide many of these nutrients by offering naturally gluten-free grains such as wholegrain rice, buckwheat and quinoa, as well as leafy green vegetables and nuts and seeds. Calcium-rich options include collard greens, other dark green leafy vegetables, bone-in fish and dairy. During the winter months you may wish to consider a vitamin-D supplement.

- **Good bacteria:** Some studies suggest that changes can occur in the type and number of beneficial bacteria present in the digestive system of children (and adults) who follow a gluten-free diet. Encourage your child to eat fermented foods, such as raw sauerkraut, kimchi, kefir, kombucha and yogurt. If your child is dairy intolerant as well as allergic to gluten, offer coconut kefir or coconut, soy or nut yogurt.
- **Iron:** To ensure sufficient iron in your child's diet, make sure you provide meals that contain good amounts of lean meat and poultry, as well as beans and lentils, egg yolks and leafy greens. Liver is a great source of iron, too (see Slow-cooked Beef Chilli, page 234). Include foods rich in vitamin C (such as red peppers, leafy greens, fresh fruit and so on) with your child's meal, as vitamin C aids iron absorption.
- **Magnesium:** Leafy greens, nuts and seeds are brilliant sources of this important mineral, which your child needs for healthy muscles and good sleep patterns, among other important functions.
- **Vitamin B12:** This important B-vitamin helps maintain nerve and blood cells, and improve energy (low levels of B12 are linked with fatigue). Good food sources include green leafy vegetables, asparagus, avocado, lean meat, eggs, beans, pulses, oranges, sunflower seeds, pistachio nuts and fish.

Shopping for your soybean-free child

The soy bean belongs to the legume family, which includes peas, beans and peanuts. Look out for hidden soy, which is a key ingredient in many processed foods, as well as readymade soups, marinades and sauces. It may even appear in chocolate products (make your own chocolates, if you're worried). On a food label, you might see "soy" or "soy lecithin E322". Soy lecithin is particularly common as an emulsifier, which stabilizes foods and stops ingredients separating. As lecithin is mainly fat rather than protein, you may find that your child can tolerate it more easily than whole soybean products. However, it is really important to check with your doctor or dietician before introducing it into your child's diet.

Soy foods to avoid	Foods to check carefully
• Edamame • Miso • Natto • Soybeans • Soy cheese • Soy flour • Soy milk and desserts, such as soy yogurt • Soy oil • Soy sauce, tamari, or teriyaki sauce • Tempeh • Textured vegetable protein (TVP) • Tofu	• Batter mixes • Breads, cakes, pizza bases and biscuits, including gluten-free products • Chocolate • Dairy-free margarines • Flavoured crisps and crackers • Ice cream • Margarine • Sausages, burgers and prepared pies • Soups • Vegetarian products – including veggie sausages, burgers and ready meals

Substituting soybean foods

Known as a key ingredient in Asian cooking, or to add flavour to homemade sauces, marinades and soups, soy sauce is a staple condiment in many kitchens. But there are lots of useful alternatives you can use when you're cooking at home.

I need a substitute for...	Try...
Soy sauce	• Brown sauce • Concentrated chicken stock • Coconut aminos • Fish sauce
Soy oil	• Cold-pressed organic rapeseed oil • Olive oil
Soy margarines	• Butter • Coconut oil • Olive-oil spread
Edamame	• Lentils • Other beans • Peas
Tofu or tempeh	• For vegetarians or vegans: use beans or pulses • For meat-eaters: use meat or fish

Soybean-free nutrition

Soybeans are an important source of complete protein, particularly for children who are being raised as vegetarians or vegans. If your child doesn't eat meat or eggs (which are also good sources of protein), make sure you include plenty other protein-rich foods, such as nuts, seeds, peas and, if they are tolerated, other beans.

Shopping for your sesame-free child

Indian, Chinese, Greek and Asian foods commonly use sesame, both in seed and oil form, in their cooking. Because of its sweet, nutty flavour, you may also find it is an ingredient in lots of desserts and pastries.

Sesame foods to avoid	Foods to check carefully
• Sesame seeds • Sesame oil • Tahini	• Breaded products • Breads, breadsticks, bagels and crackers • Chocolate bars and sweets • Dips, salad dressings and sauces, especially Greek dips such as hummus and babaganoush, Asian stir-fry sauces and Indian curry sauces • Falafels • Margarines and spreads • Middle Eastern sweets and pastries • Muesli, granola, breakfast cereals and cereal bars (including flapjacks) • Veggie burgers and sausages

Substituting sesame

Sesame one of the easiest allergen foods to substitute, because in fact any nut or seed oil, or whole seed will work just as well. Light olive oils makes a good alternative if nuts and seeds are generally off the menu for your child.

I need a substitute for...	Try...
Sesame oil	In dips and dressings: • Any non-allergen nut or seed oil • Cold pressed rapeseed oil • Light olive oil In Asian cooking: • Miso paste • Tamari sauce

I need a substitute for...	Try...
Tahini	Any non-allergen nut or seed butter
Sesame seeds	Any non-allergen seeds

Sesame-free nutrition

Not only are sesame seeds an excellent source of copper and a very good source of manganese, they are also a good source of calcium and magnesium (for bone health), iron, phosphorus, vitamin B1, zinc, molybdenum, selenium and dietary fibre. Many of these nutrients are important for the immune system and for the body's energy production. You can find many of these nutrients in other foods, including other nuts and seeds if your child can tolerate them.

Shopping for your sulphite-free child

Sulphites consist of a group of sulphur-based chemicals, including sulphur dioxide (SO2). They are essentially food preservatives (you may see them listed on labels as E numbers from E220 to E228) that manufacturers use to prevent foods going brown or in other ways discolouring. Sulphur dioxide has to appear on labels when the food product contains more than 10mg/kg or 10mg per litre.

E-numbers to avoid	Foods to check carefully
• E220 (Sulphur dioxide) • E221 (Sodium sulphite) • E222 (Sodium hydrogen sulphite) • E223 (Sodium metabisulphite) • E224 (Potassium metabisulphite) • E226 (Calcium sulphite) • E227 (Calcium hydrogen sulphite) • E228 (Potassium hydrogen sulphite)	• Dried fruit and vegetables • Frozen potato products • Frozen seafood, such as prawns and shrimp • Fruit yogurts • Jams and other preserves • Pickles, vinegars and bottled lemon juice • Sausages and cured meats • Soft drinks, including fruit juices • Stock cubes and processed gravies

Substituting sulphites

Interestingly, a supplement containing vitamin C and E may reduce a child's sensitivity to sulphur dioxide, making substitutions easier to handle. Consult your doctor or dietician before trying this, though, and proceed only under medical advice. In general, it is possible to find sulphite-free versions of most products, but they are not always easy to source. Avoiding or reducing your child's intake of sulphites is not likely to cause any nutritional deficiencies.

For a child who is sulphite free, seek out fresh foods (unpackaged) over frozen or dried, as this way you can be fairly certain you're avoiding sulphites. Instead of fruit yogurts, use organic, natural yogurt and flavour it with pieces of fresh fruit, or make your own purées to stir through.

I need a substitute for...	Try...
Vinegar	• Fresh lemon juice
Shop-bought dressings or jams	• A homemade dressing of cold-pressed seed or nut oils or olive oil mixed with fresh lemon juice • Homemade jams
Fruit juice drinks	• Squeeze your own orange juice or make smoothies of fresh fruit and vegetables • Organic, fresh bought juices
Dried or frozen fruit and vegetables	• Unbagged fresh fruit and vegetables • Sulphite-free organic dried fruit or vegetables
Stock cubes and processed gravies	• Homemade bone broth (see page 190) • Organic brands, which are usually sulphite free

Shopping for your shellfish-free child

For labelling purposes, shellfish is divided into two categories (see below). Even if your child is allergic to one type and not the other, you will need to be extremely careful to avoid cross-contamination as different types of shellfish are often found together on fish counters or are processed and packaged in the same factory.

- crustacea (including prawn, lobster, crab, crayfish, langoustine and scampi)
- molluscs (periwinkles, whelks, mussels, scallops, clams, oysters, octopus, squid and cockles)

- when reading the labels, the product should be clearly highlighted either as crustacea or mollusc

In addition to shellfish itself, watch out for the following, which may contain shellfish:

- fish stocks and soups
- paella
- pasta sauces (even tomato sauce can contain fish or shellfish sauce)
- oriental fish sauces and sauces such as bisque
- Indian and Thai curry pastes

Also bear in mind that sushi may be contaminated even it's made using fish rather than shellfish. And be mindful of foods that may have been dipped in the same batter or cooked in the same oil as shellfish foods (for example, chips may be fried in the same oil as scampi). Be aware that some supplements may contain shellfish.

Substituting shellfish

Other fish, if tolerated, as well as meat, poultry, eggs, beans and pulses, or tofu are all good substitutes for shellfish. Instead of fish sauce and oyster sauce, use gluten-free tamari soy sauce or miso paste. You can replace shellfish-containing fish stocks with homemade bone broth (see page 190), chicken or vegetable stocks.

Shellfish-free nutrition

While shellfish is an excellent source of protein, healthy fats and key vitamins and minerals (including B-vitamins, zinc, iron, selenium, potassium and magnesium), other protein-rich foods, including fish, are also good sources of all these nutrients. Shellfish is also a useful source of iodine, which is often low in the diets of both children and adults. Iodine is important for metabolism, thyroid function and brain health, and growth and development in children. Other iodine sources include sea vegetables (you can buy dried sea-vegetable mixes and add them to soups or stews), cranberries, organic yogurt and cheese. Try also using sea-vegetable salt mixes as a flavouring in recipes. Eggs, fish (such as cod and tuna), prunes and green peas are also good sources of iodine.

Shopping for your fish-free child

If your child is allergic to fish, you will need to read labels very carefully – in particular, many condiments and sauces include fish stock, fish sauce, or anchovies as a flavouring. Even if only certain types of fish have been identified as culprit foods for your child (your doctor or allergy specialist should be able to specify), there is always a high risk of cross-contamination. For example, one type of fish may become contaminated during the catching process, or transportation, or packaging, or once it reaches a fishmonger counter.

While some forms of fish or shellfish may be visible in food, other forms may be hidden, or not obvious by sight or smell. The following list of foods commonly contain "hidden" fish:

- dips or pâtés such as taramasalata, caviar or roe (fish eggs)
- dressings and toppings, such as those in Caesar salads or on pizzas (both of which often contain anchovies)
- marshmallows and nougat, which may contain fish-based gelatine
- rice dishes such as paella, fried rice and sushi rolls

- sauces and condiments, including Worcestershire sauce
- stews, soups or casseroles, such as chowder or bouillabaisse

Be aware that some supplements may be derived from fish or may be processed in the same factory as other supplements containing fish. While most fish-oil supplements are processed to remove the proteins that typically trigger an allergic reaction, your child may still react. Speak to your child's allergy specialist before choosing an omega-3 supplement, and aim always to look for vegan-based supplements in general.

Substituting fish

Other proteins, including meat, poultry, eggs, beans and pulses or tofu are all good substitutes for fish. Instead of fish sauce, use gluten-free tamari soy sauce or miso paste.

Fish-free nutrition

Fish, particularly oily fish (salmon, sardines, mackerel, anchovies and so on), is an excellent source of protein and anti-inflammatory omega-3 fats. It also provides a range of vitamins and minerals including vitamins B2 and D, calcium, phosphorus, iron, zinc, iodine, magnesium and potassium.

Omega-3 fats are crucial for the health of your child's developing brain and nervous system. They also lower inflammation in the body, and contribute to good eye health. To ensure a fish-free child gains ample amounts of omega-3 fats, consider a vegan supplement (made using algae sources) and offer your child daily portions of seeds, such as flaxseed, chia and pumpkin, as well as walnuts, tofu and leafy greens. You can also try using cold-pressed flaxseed oil in dressings (never heat this kind of oil, though, as it is easily damaged during cooking). If your child can tolerate shellfish, and as long as you are mindful of cross-contamination, this is another great way to provide omega-3s in the diet. Non-fish sources of vitamin D include liver and eggs, but consider a supplement, too (see page 145).

Shopping for your mustard-free child

It is not just jars of mustard you would need to be mindful of if your child has a mustard allergy. Mustard seeds are often added to salad dressings, curry pastes and prepared sauces (including barbecue, béchamel, hollandaise, mayonnaise and salad cream), as well as to stocks, soups and ready meals. Mustard is often used as a flavouring in sausages, burgers and Indian curries, and the seeds are often sprinkled over bread rolls and used in naan breads. Look out for dishes containing mustard leaves, too (this is particularly important for Asian foods).

Substituting mustard

The best way to avoid mustard is to use your own homemade bone broth (see page 190) and flavour with herbs and individual spices rather than using mixed spices or shop-bought stock cubes. Most recipes will work just as well if you leave out mustard powder or mustard sauce, but if you need a strong flavouring, try horseradish, pure wasabi paste, caraway seeds or turmeric.

Mustard-free nutrition

While mustard seeds are a useful source of certain nutrients, such as selenium, the amount in a dish is so small that avoiding mustard will not contribute to any significant deficiencies in an otherwise healthy and varied diet.

Shopping for your celery-free child

Celery stems, leaves and seeds (the latter are often in spice and herbs mixes and packet seasonings) are all useable parts of the plant and may appear in recipes and ready-made foods. In the latter case, always check the labels (particularly for shop-bought soups and stews, and coleslaws which often contain celery or celery seeds). Note that the root vegetable celeriac is closely related to celery, so if your child has a celery allergy, make sure you avoid that, too.

In particular look out for celery as an ingredient in stock cubes and bouillon powder, gravy, soups, sauces, stews, salads, tomato juice, spice mixes, crisps and also Marmite.

Substituting celery

The best way to avoid celery is to cook using your own home-made stock (see page 000) and flavour your dishes with individual herbs and spices. In recipes, instead of celery seeds, try fennel or caraway seeds.

Celery-free nutrition

While celery is an excellent source of many antioxidants, vitamin K, and molybdenum, providing your child with a wide variety of vegetables, including leafy greens, will provide sufficient quantities of these nutrients in his or her diet.

Shopping for your lupin-free child

If your child is allergic to lupin be mindful that some gluten-free products may contain lupin flour as a substitute for wheat flour. Look out for baked goods, including breads, pizza bases, and pastries, as well as pancakes, waffles, crumbed foods (including fried foods such as onion rings), pastas, flour mixes, sausages and burgers.

Substituting lupin

Lupin is not commonly used in recipes, so is easy to avoid – using flour mixes that don't contain this legume is all you need to do.

Lupin-free nutrition

Lupin, like many legumes, is a good source of fibre, protein and various B-vitamins, as well as minerals such as manganese, copper,

Lupin

The lupin plant is part of the legume family alongside peanuts and peas. A number of studies demonstrate that those with a peanut allergy are also more susceptible to a lupin allergy, so consult your child's doctor or allergy specialist if you're concerned. Incidences of lupin allergy are relatively uncommon in the UK; in other countries, such as France and elsewhere on mainland Europe, where lupin seeds or beans are often crushed to make flour, the incidences are higher. A child who is allergic to lupin as a food may come up with a skin rash or other allergic symptom if he or she were to handle the seeds of the garden flower. Check your garden for lupins (they are tall finger-like stems covered with purple or pink flowers) and remove them if there is a risk your child might touch or play with them.

Yeast overgrowth

Children, like adults, have naturally occurring yeasts in their bodies – notably in the mouth and intestines. An overgrowth of yeast, such as *Candida albicans*, in the body can lead to symptoms such as skin rashes, oral thrush, recurrent ear infections and headaches, among others. The overgrowth often occurs when there is an imbalance of gut flora. If you suspect your child has a yeast infection, ask your doctor for a stool test to confirm the diagnosis. Then, if it's positive, take steps to eradicate the yeast growth, including by reducing his or her sugar intake (sugar is yeast food!).

magnesium, phosphorus, potassium and zinc. However, a varied diet that includes other beans and pulses (if tolerated), as well as meat, fish, eggs, nuts, seeds and a host of vegetables will mean that your child has plenty of other super-sources of these vital nutrients.

Beyond the 14 allergens: yeast

Although in the UK and EU, the Food Standards Agency has identified 14 key allergens, there are, of course, many more. One that I particularly want to mention is yeast, a living fungus that is an active ingredient (a catalyst of sorts) in many different foods.

In general, a child who reacts to yeast (both brewer's yeast and baker's yeast) has a food sensitivity rather than an IgE-mediated food allergy (see page 23). A child with a yeast sensitivity may also react to mushrooms, blue cheeses and malt. When reading labels look out for the terms hydrolysed protein, hydrolysed vegetable protein, or leavening. These are all indications that yeast is likely to be present in the food.

Yeast foods to avoid	Foods to treat with caution
• Beer, wine, ciders (including those used in cooking) • Dried fruit • Fermented foods, such as sauerkraut, miso • Fermented health drinks, such as kombucha • Ginger beer • Gravy and stock cubes • Marmite or Vegemite • Mushrooms • Sweet breads or cakes, such as doughnuts, muffins, Chelsea buns, teacakes, brioche and croissants • Vinegar (including vinaigrettes, pickles and chutneys) • Yeasted breads, including sourdough, pizza bases and bread rolls (but not soda bread)	• Nuts and seeds, which may be contaminated with moulds • Quorn

Substituting yeast foods

For flavourings and dressings, use fresh citrus juice instead of vinegar. Soda bread is naturally yeast free, so makes a perfect alternative to yeasted breads. It's also really easy to make savoury crackers, pizza bases and muffins without the need for yeast. Rice cakes, oat cakes and so on make useful substitutes for yeasted crackers and bread snacks. Stock cubes are difficult to replace, but most stores now sell freshly prepared stock, or you can make your own (see page 190). Some vegetable bouillon powders are yeast free – so check labels while you're shopping and see what's available. Adding a dash of toasted sesame oil or fish sauce to soups and stews can add extra flavour in place of stock, if you prefer.

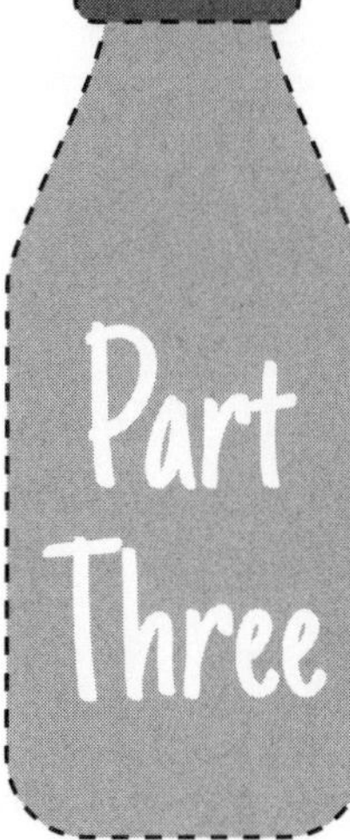

Mealtimes in practice

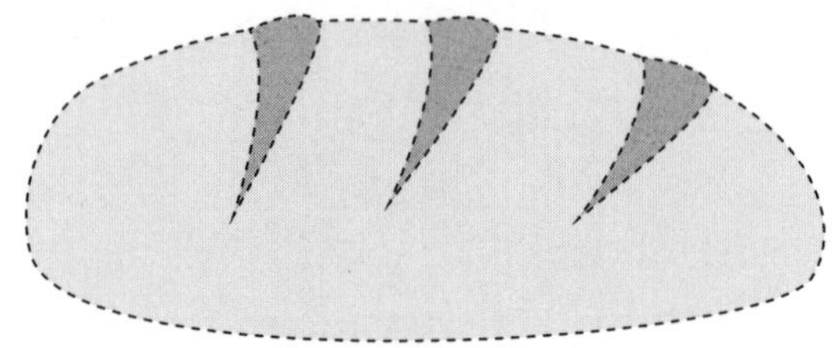

Eating well is fundamental to good health, growth and development and can be a powerful tool in helping to improve immune function and gut health, which are key players when it comes to allergies. Eating should also be an enjoyable, sociable experience for children and adults alike. Studies prove that establishing healthy eating patterns during childhood helps promote healthier habits long term.

Feeding an active child with healthy, nourishing food that they want to eat and you have time to make can be tricky at the best of times, but add to that the need to avoid certain foods and mealtimes are trickier still. The recipes in this book are designed to help you feed your whole family with delicious, easy and nourishing meals that also happen to be allergy free. Rather than cooking separate food for your child, these recipes are perfect for everyone.

Building your meals

The most important thing to think about when building meals for your family is balance.

- Ideally half of the plate should be a range of colourful vegetables (raw or cooked) – and feel free to use frozen vegetables for speed. Aim for two or three servings of vegetables at main meals, and don't forget you can get vegetables in even at breakfast – try grilled mushrooms and tomatoes with scrambled egg or scrambled tofu; or try adding a handful of spinach to a fruity kefir smoothie.
- Fill a quarter of the plate with protein-rich foods, such as lean meats, fish, poultry, beans and pulses, tofu, tempeh or edamame beans, dairy-free yogurt and cheese alternatives.
- Fill the remaining quarter with some slow-releasing carbohydrates, such as starchy vegetables (for example, sweet potato, swede, carrot, beetroot or potato) or whole grains (such as wholegrain rice or quinoa).
- Add healthy fats, perhaps as a dressing (using healthy oils, such as olive, avocado, flaxseed or walnut), or a sprinkling of nuts and seeds, or avocado slices, or a handful of olives.
- Try to make sure that your meals include gut-healthy options: try the apple sauerkraut recipe on page 197, or make it into coleslaw; use dairy-free kefir, dairy-free yogurts, and miso.

Making meals count

Blood-sugar balance is so important for children, regardless of whether or not they have an allergy, and that means trying to ensure that they have a steady stream of energy throughout the day – not energy peaks and troughs. Healthy meals that supply constant energy, topped up with healthy snacks if needed, mean that children are far less likely to demand unhealthy, sugar-rich snacks. Remember that sugar has an inflammatory effect on the body, disrupts the balance of gut flora and upsets immune function. Try not to let your child graze throughout the day, and instead encourage three meals and one or two nutritious snacks, if needed. It's important to make snacks count nutritionally. Avoid empty calories, such as crisps, cakes, fizzy drinks, sweets and so on. There are lots of snack recipes in the book, as well as the easy suggestions in the box opposite.

A rough guide to portion sizes

Age and activity levels will influence how much your child needs to eat – more active children are more likely to need snacks as well as meals, and there will be certain times during growth spurts when you feel that you can't feed your children enough. As a very rough guide, teenagers are likely to need similar portions to adults (see below). For primary school children, use half the amount.

Each of these represents a single portion as part of a full meal:

- 100g/3½oz leafy greens (raw)
- 80g/2¾oz other vegetables
- Starchy vegetables: ½ sweet potato or ½ baked potato
- 65g/2¼oz (cooked weight) gluten-free grains
- Fruit: 1 small apple (about 80g/2¾oz)

Easy nutritious snacks

The following snacks are all super-nutritious and easy to rustle up for hungry, active children. Use these as well as the nutritious snacks that I've included in the recipe section of the book.

- Brioche-style bread (see page 186), seeded bread (see page 188) or gluten-free bread spread with hummus, guacamole (see page 283), seed or nut butters, canned fish and so on
- Dairy-free plain yogurt with fruit
- Fresh fruit slices with nut or seed butter
- Cooked slices of chicken, turkey, beef and so on
- Cooked prawns
- Smoked salmon slices
- Hard-boiled eggs
- Toasted seeds and nuts
- Olives
- Spicy chickpeas (see page 284)
- Raw vegetables, such as carrots, peppers, cherry tomatoes, cucumber or celery, with dips such as hummus or dairy-free yogurt, fish pâté or guacamole
- Homemade popcorn
- Gluten-free crackers or oatcakes, rice cakes or buckwheat seed crackers (see page 280) spread with nut or seed butter or other protein spreads
- Homemade vegetable and berry smoothies

- 100g/3½oz (uncooked weight) lean meat like beef, lamb or pork
- 100g/3½oz (uncooked weight) fish
- 2 eggs
- 75g/2¾oz beans (cooked)
- 30g/1oz nuts
- 100g/3½oz/scant ½ cup dairy-free yogurt
- 250ml/9fl oz/generous 1 cup dairy-free milk

Make time for breakfast

Children who miss breakfast become hungry and tired, which can affect their concentration and performance at school or in other tasks. This goes for every child, whether or not he or she has an allergy. What's particularly important for children with allergies, though, especially while they are still little is that feeling hungry may lead to temptation to eat unhealthy foods as a quick fix. In order to optimize your child's diet and maintain balanced gut health, foods that are high in sugar and are processed are especially off the menu. A healthy breakfast, rich in protein, will be sustaining for a morning of activity and keeping risky temptation at bay.

Allergy-sensitive packed lunches

Creating a healthy packed lunch may be the best way to ensure that children with food allergies have allergen-free food to eat while they are at school or otherwise away from home. All the principles of providing a balanced, nutritious meal apply to packed lunches, too. There are a couple of things that are especially worth mentioning, though, if you have a child with allergies:

- **Dairy-free options:** It is generally recommended that you include some calcium-rich food in your child's packed lunch and, for most children, one of the easiest options is often dairy. If your child has to avoid dairy, you can still include calcium-rich foods by packing homemade fruit smoothies made with fortified milk alternatives; serve a small pot of dairy-free plain yogurt with fruit on the side or mixed in; include canned sardines or salmon in salads or sandwiches; use tahini or almond nut butter as a spread, or stir them into dips such as hummus. You can also pack some toasted seeds (sesame, poppy, chia, sunflower or pumpkin), or use cooked beans and lentils or cooked tofu in salads. Look for fortified breads when making sandwiches.
- **Starchy carbs:** Whole grains and starchy vegetables, such as sweet potato, beetroot, carrots and peas, are all great options for supporting your child's energy, as well as providing fibre for digestive health, which is so important for immune balance. To make a change from sandwiches, try wholegrain rice or quinoa in a salad, or make use of soba or rice noodles. Serve gluten-free crackers, rice cakes, or buckwheat crackers on the side with some lean protein or dips. Sweet potato wedges, corn tortillas, corn chips, popcorn and gluten-free oat cakes are all great portable options.

With dairy and carbs sorted, be sure to include healthy protein, plenty of vegetables and a little fruit (think colour), and a bottle of water. Water is by far the most healthy drink for children regardless of their allergy status. Flavour it with a slice of cucumber, or lemon or lime, if you wish.

The packed lunch week

Use these ideas to create variety in your child's packed lunches over the course of a week.

Monday

- Green smoothie (blend a banana, a handful of spinach, 150ml/5fl oz coconut water and 100ml/3½fl oz dairy-free milk)
- Carrot and cucumber slices
- Cooked chicken slices
- Rice cakes or buckwheat seed crackers (see page 280)
- Apple wedges

Tuesday

- Gluten-free pitta with homemade meatballs (see page 241) or Falafel bites with salsa and minted dip (see page 222)
- Cherry tomatoes
- Vegetable crisps (see page 282)
- Fruit salad

Wednesday

- Homemade pasty (see page 224)
- Red pepper and carrot sticks
- Berry kefir shake (see page 199)

Thursday

- Rice, salmon and vegetable salad
- Ginger oaty cookie (see page 286)
- Satsuma

Friday

- Roast beef and sauerkraut gluten-free wrap (see sandwich-filler recipes)
- Baby sweetcorn and mangetout
- Strawberries and dairy-free yogurt

Sample week meal plans

The following tables use recipes in the book to create sample meal plans for two different allergen-free weeks, and a week of boosting the immune system and restoring gut health. Remember that all the recipes in the book are gluten free (as long as shopbought ingredients are certified gluten free, too). Use these representative weeks to get you started, then mix and match to create a healthy and varied diet for your entire family – one that everyone, no matter what allergies they have, can enjoy.

Gluten- and dairy-free sample week

DAY	BREAKFAST	LUNCH
Monday	Fruity millet porridge (see p.207) with berries, nuts and seeds	Gluten-free pitta with falafel bites (see p.222) Cherry tomatoes and cucumber slices Fruit salad with dairy-free yogurt
Tuesday	Breakfast seed bar (see p.208) Berry kefir shake (see p.200)	Leftover cornbread (see p.236) Hard-boiled egg or pot of hummus Vegetable sticks Piece of fruit
Wednesday	Scrambled eggs with smoked salmon and spinach	Mexican taco chicken salad with avocado dressing (see p.229) Breakfast seed bar (see p.208) Piece of fruit
Thursday	Baked beans on waffles (see p.211)	Leftover barbecue traybake chicken (see p.245) Rice cakes Cucumber and carrot slices Apple wedges
Friday	Dairy-free yogurt with carrot cake granola (see p.201)	Leftover smoky bean burgers (see p.264) with gluten-free roll Fruity coleslaw (see p.247) Berry kefir shake (see p.200)
Saturday	Salmon kedgeree (see p.213)	Chicken noodle soup (see p.218) Salad Tropical parfait (see p.272)
Sunday	American pancakes with berry compôte (see p.203)	Pineapple and pork salad (see p.225) Speedy banana ice cream (see p.269)

DINNER	SNACKS
Slow-cooked beef chilli (see p.234) with steamed vegetables Cornbread (see p.236) Tropical parfait (see p.272)	Hummus with vegetable sticks
Fish bites with homemade tomato ketchup (see p.255) Mixed salad Peas and carrots Berry apple crumble (see p.275)	Apple slices with nut or seed butter or dairy-free yogurt
Barbecue traybake chicken (see p.245) Salad and fruity coleslaw (see p.247) Fruit slices	Carrot cake granola (see p.201) with dairy-free yogurt
Smoky bean burgers (see p.264) Mixed salad and leftover coleslaw (see p.231) Steamed vegetables Speedy banana ice cream (see p.269)	Apple streusel muffin (see p.205)
Chowder fish pie (see p.253) with steamed vegetables and salad Fruit with dairy-free yogurt	Vegetable crisps (see p.282) Hard-boiled egg
Chunky veg stew with herby dumplings (see p.262) Salad Gooey lemon dessert (see p.278)	Creamy guacamole (see p.283) with vegetable sticks or Buckwheat seed crackers (see p.280)
Creamy prawn tikka masala (see p.257) with wholegrain rice	Satsuma Spicy chickpeas (see p.284)

Egg-, gluten- and dairy-free sample week

DAY	BREAKFAST	LUNCH
Monday	Carrot cake granola (see p.201) with berries and dairy-free yogurt	Gluten-free cocktail sausages Buckwheat seed crackers (see p.280) Cherry tomatoes, olives and cucumber slices Fruit salad
Tuesday	Berry kefir shake (see p.200) Breakfast seed bar (see p.208)	Rice paper rolls (see p.220) Carrot sticks Apple streusel muffin (see p.205) Pot of blueberries
Wednesday	Fruity millet porridge (see p.207) with apricots	Slice of leftover pizza (see p.227) Fruity coleslaw (see p.247) Cucumber slices Piece of fruit
Thursday	Baked beans on gluten-free bread	Leftover sweet potato and salmon fish cakes (see p.259) Homemade tomato ketchup (see p.255) Vegetable sticks Berry kefir shake (see p.200)
Friday	Leftover rice pudding with spiced plum compôte (see p.276) and dairy-free yogurt	Mexican taco chicken salad with avocado dressing (see p.229) Fruit salad
Saturday	Breakfast sweet potato chorizo hash (see p.210)	Roasted red pepper tortilla soup (see p.216) Salad with cooked chicken slices Fresh fruit
Sunday	Tropical parfait (see p.272)	Fish bites with homemade tomato ketchup (see page 255) Salad Dairy-free yogurt with berries

DINNER	SNACK
Chowder fish pie (see p.253) Steamed vegetables and salad Speedy banana ice cream (see p.269)	Satsuma Spicy chickpeas (see p.284)
Pizza (see p.227) with salad and homemade fruity coleslaw (see p.247) Steamed vegetables and salad Easy chocolate mousse (see p.273)	Ginger oaty cookie (see p.286)
Sweet potato and salmon fish cakes (see p.259) with fruity coleslaw (see p.247), sweet potato wedges and vegetables Fruit salad	Buckwheat seed crackers (see p.280) with nut butter
Fruity lamb tagine (see p.239) Steamed vegetables Baked rice pudding with spiced plum compôte (see p.276) and dairy-free yogurt	Vegetable crisps (see p.282) Handful of granola or nuts
Harissa tray-bake vegetables and chickpeas with herby yogurt (see p.266) Berry apple crumble (see p.275) and dairy-free yogurt	Creamy guacamole (see p.283) with vegetable sticks or rice cakes
Moroccan one-pot chicken with rice (see p.249) Salad Speedy banana ice cream (see p.269)	Breakfast seed bar (see p.208)
Pulled jerk pork (see page 243) Salad and steamed vegetables Sweet potato wedges Easy chocolate mousse (see page 273)	Spicy chickpeas (see page 284) Vegetable sticks

Immune-system modulating and gut-healthy sample week

DAY	BREAKFAST	LUNCH
Monday	Carrot cake granola (see p.201) with dairy-free yogurt and berries	Mexican taco chicken salad with avocado dressing (see p.229) Ginger oaty cookie (see p.286) Berry kefir shake (see p.200)
Tuesday	Leftover chilli	Falafel bites with salsa and minted dip (see p.221) in gluten free pitta Dairy-free yogurt with sliced fruit
Wednesday	Berry kefir shake (see p.200) Carrot cake granola (see p.201) with berries	Leftover sweet potato and salmon fish cakes (see p.259) Fruity coleslaw (see p.247) Cherry tomatoes Piece of fruit
Thursday	Tropical parfait (see p.272)	Buckwheat seed crackers (see p.280) Pot of hummus or sliced barbecue chicken Vegetable sticks Piece of fruit
Friday	American pancakes with berry compôte (see p.203)	Salmon and cucumber gluten-free wrap (see p.231) Olives and cherry tomatoes Fruit salad
Saturday	Salmon kedgeree (see p.213)	Breakfast bean burritos (see p.209) Creamy guacamole (see p.283) Salad Fruit
Sunday	Berry kefir shake (see p.200) Breakfast sweet potato hash (see p.210)	Chicken noodle soup (see p.218) with salad Fresh fruit salad and yogurt

DINNER	SNACK
Slow-cooked beef chilli (see p.234) with Cornbread (see p.236) and salad Speedy banana ice cream (see p.269)	Apple sauerkraut (see p.197) with buckwheat seed crackers (see p.280) or rice cakes
Sweet potato and salmon fish cakes (see p.259) Fruity coleslaw (see p.247) Salad Berry kefir shake (see p.200)	Vegetable crisps (see p.282) Apple with nut butter
Harissa tray-bake vegetables and chickpeas with herby yogurt (see p.266) Salad Fruit salad and dairy-free yogurt	Hard-boiled egg Rice cakes
Pesto meatball pasta bake (see p.241) Easy chocolate mousse (see p.273)	Carrot cake granola (see p.201) with dairy-free yogurt
Chicken schnitzel with coleslaw (see p.247) Berry apple crumble (see p.275) with dairy-free yogurt	Creamy guacamole (see p.283) with vegetable sticks and rice cakes
Chow mein (see p.237) Salad Speedy banana ice cream (see p.269)	Berry kefir shake (see p.200)
Chowder fish pie (see p.253) with salad Strawberry jam mug cake (see p.274) with dairy-free yogurt	Breakfast seed bar (see p.208)

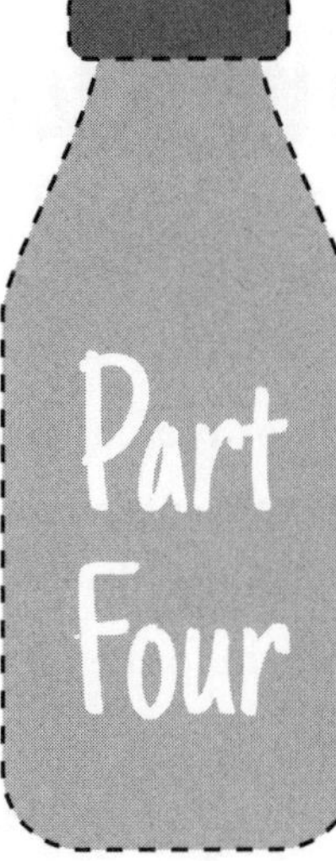

Recipes

A Note on the Recipes

Food intolerances should not prevent anyone from eating tasty and varied meals. My own experiences have led me to create recipes for children affected by allergies that they (and their parents) will enjoy. In addition, all the dishes are nutrient rich to help support a healthy immune response and gut healing. The focus of this book is on child-friendly food while reducing, as far as possible, the use of refined sugar, which is linked to hyperactivity as well as obesity and other long-term health problems. Instead, I favour xylitol, erythritol or stevia which, unlike refined sugar, do not have a high calorific content or create swings in blood sugar levels. You will however need to use regular sugar in recipes for bread, as it is the sugar that feeds the yeast. Occasionally, in cooking, I use a little liquid sweetener such as honey or maple syrup, but I only use these in very small amounts.

All recipes are gluten free and dairy free. For each recipe there is a key at the side of each page to indicate at a glance those that are suitable for vegetarians or vegans, as well as dishes that are egg, nut or soy free. (For the purposes of identifying ingredients that may cause a reaction I am classing coconut as a nut because although coconut is actually a fruit not a nut, some people who are allergic to tree nuts (for example, almonds, cashews and walnuts) also react to coconut. Not everyone is affected; it's wise to check with your GP if your child has a nut allergy.) Where a recipe key note appears in brackets, you need to make sure that you are using the correct free-from alternative to avoid an ingredient that affects your child. Dairy-free milk and spreads, for example, may be made from nuts or soy. Always check the labels of products you buy to ensure that you are not inadvertently including gluten or dairy products; for example, certain brands of baking powder or mayonnaise may contain these. There are now branded products that replace, for instance, eggs where they are used as thickeners but I also suggest ways you can make your own alternative and still get excellent results.

Basics

While you can purchase gluten-free flour blends it is easy to make your own. Here are a couple of easy blends that you can make up and store in an airtight container ready for use in recipes. Don't forget to label the mixes.

Gluten-free flour blend for cookies, pastry and pancakes/waffles

350g/12oz/3½ cups fine white rice or brown rice flour
100g/3½oz/1 cup potato flour
50g/2oz/½ cup tapioca flour

Gluten-free bread flour blend

400g/14oz/4 cups buckwheat flour, brown rice flour or sorghum flour
200g/7oz/2 cups tapioca flour
400g/14oz/4 cups potato flour
300g/10½oz/3 cups cornflour/cornstarch

When baking with your own gluten-free flour mixes you may need to add a little xanthum gum to help bind the mixture – this will depend on the recipe and whether other binders like eggs are also being used. However, as a general guide, if it is not already included in your flour blend, mix 2 tsp of xanthum gum per 500g/1lb 2oz/5 cups gluten-free flour mix for bread and ¼ tsp per 200g/7oz/2 cups flour for cakes. Using too much xanthan gum can make your baking a little heavy, so experiment with a small amount – say ¼ tsp – first. If you want to create a self-raising/self-rising flour mix, simply add 25g gluten-free baking powder per 500g/1lb 2oz/5 cups of flour mix.

Shortcrust Pastry/Pie Dough

Makes 450g/1lb pastry/pie dough

Vegetarian
(Nut Free)
(Soy Free)

This is such an easy gluten-free, dairy-free pastry and it can be used for both sweet and savoury dishes. The trick with gluten-free pastry is to make sure the dough is slightly on the moist side because if it is too dry it will crumble when you roll it. For ease, roll it between sheets of cling film/plastic wrap. You can store the pastry dough in the refrigerator for 2–3 days or freeze for 1 month.

Preparation time: 15 minutes
Chilling time: 30 minutes

360g/12oz/3¼ cups gluten-free flour blend (see page 182)
¼ tsp sea salt
1 tsp xanthum gum
175g/6oz dairy-free spread, chilled and cut into small pieces
1 egg, beaten
3 tbsp cold water to blend

1 Put the flour, salt, and xanthum gum in a food processor and briefly process. Alternatively mix them together in a bowl.
2 Add the chilled dairy-free spread and process to form breadcrumbs or rub in using your fingers.
3 Add the beaten egg and process or combine with sufficient water to form a soft dough. It should be slightly damp.
4 Form into a ball and flatten to form a circle. Wrap in cling film/plastic wrap then chill for at least 30 minutes, which makes it easier to roll.
5 When you are ready to use the pastry, place the dough between two sheets of cling film/plastic wrap. Roll out to the required thickness.

Corn Tortillas

Makes 4–6 tortillas

Vegetarian
Vegan
Egg Free
Nut Free
Soy Free

These golden tortillas only require a handful of ingredients and make a change from bread. Traditionally they are made using a naturally gluten-free maize flour, masa harina, which is very different from standard cornflour/cornstarch and has a distinctive gold colour. Masa harina is available from supermarkets, health food shops and online. However, you can also use a mixture of fine polenta/cornmeal and gluten-free flour. Roll out the dough thinly so that the tortillas can be rolled or folded once cooked.

Preparation time: 15 minutes
Cooking time: 16 minutes

300g/10½oz/2⅔ cups masa harina flour (or 50:50 fine polenta/cornmeal and gluten-free bread flour), plus extra for rolling
1 tsp sea salt
1 tsp xanthan gum
1 tsp gluten-free baking powder
250ml/9fl oz/1 cup warm water
olive oil, for brushing

1 Put the flour, salt and xanthan gum in a large bowl or food processor and gradually add enough water and process or combine until you have a firm, slightly damp dough.
2 Place a large piece of cling film/plastic wrap on the work surface and dust with a little gluten-free flour.
3 Divide the dough into four equal pieces and place one piece on the cling film/plastic wrap, coating both sides with the flour. Roll out with a rolling pin to form a round about 2–3mm/⅛in thick. Using a bowl or plate about 15cm/6in diameter as a

guide, cut out a neat round. Set aside and repeat with the remaining dough.

4 When ready to cook, lightly oil a crêpe or shallow frying pan. Heat the pan until hot then place a circle of dough in the pan. Brush the top side with a little more oil. Allow the tortilla to cook for 1–2 minutes until lightly golden underneath. Flip over and cook for another minute. Repeat with the remaining tortillas. Once cooled these can be frozen and later reheated in the oven or microwave.

Makes 1 loaf/about 10 slices

Brioche-style Loaf

Vegetarian
(Egg Free)
(Nut Free)
(Soy Free)

This is a rich bread, perfect as a breakfast or brunch treat and equally delicious sliced for sandwiches. This version uses far less sugar than traditional recipes and is also dairy free. It will keep in the fridge for 2–3 days or you can freeze it for up to 3 months.

For an egg-free bread add an extra 4 tbsp dairy-free milk and an extra 1 tbsp olive oil in place of the eggs.

Preparation time: 15 minutes plus proving time
Cooking time: 45 minutes

200ml/7fl oz/scant 1 cup dairy-free milk
2 x 7g sachets fast-action/instant active dried yeast
2 tbsp caster/superfine sugar
500g/1lb 2oz/5 cups gluten-free bread flour blend (or for recipe see page 182)
1 tsp xanthum gum
1 tsp gluten-free baking powder
½ tsp sea salt
175ml/6fl oz/¾ cup carbonated water
60g/2½oz melted dairy-free spread or olive oil
2 eggs, beaten

1 If using a bread machine, simply place all the ingredients into the lightly oiled loaf pan in the order listed and stir briefly. Select a sweet bread option and start the machine.
2 To make the bread without a machine, warm the milk to lukewarm. Stir in the yeast and sugar and allow it to froth for 10 minutes.

3 Put the flour, xanthum gum, baking powder and salt into the bowl of a mixer fitted with a dough hook. Add the carbonated water, dairy-free spread and eggs, followed by the yeast mixture and beat for at least 5 minutes to form a soft dough.
4 Scrape the dough into a greased bowl, cover with cling film/plastic wrap and allow it to prove for 1 hour.
5 Lightly grease a 900g/2lb loaf pan. Tip the dough into the loaf pan. Allow to prove for 30 minutes.
6 Preheat the oven to 200°C/400°F/gas mark 6. Bake the loaf for 40–45 minutes until golden and firm or until a skewer inserted into the middle comes out clean.
7 Leave to cool on a wire/cooling rack before serving.

Vegan Buckwheat Seed Bread

Makes 1 loaf/about 10 slices

Vegetarian
Vegan
Egg Free
Soy Free

This gluten-free bread is so easy to make and much higher in protein thanks to the addition of buckwheat and seeds. It is also yeast free. It's best served on the day it is made but it can be sliced and frozen, too. Remember to soak the buckwheat the night before you make this tasty bread.

Preparation time: 10 minutes
Soaking time: overnight
Cooking time: 50 minutes

75g/3oz/¾ cup buckwheat, soaked overnight then rinsed
50g/2oz/½ cup ground sunflower seeds
25g/¾oz ground flaxseed
30g/1oz/scant ½ cup coconut flour
50g/2oz/½ cup chia seeds
1 tsp bicarbonate of soda/baking soda
1 tsp gluten-free baking powder
½ tsp xanthum gum
300ml/10½ fl oz/1¼ cups water
1 tbsp olive oil
2 tsp powdered psyllium husks
½ tsp sea salt
1 tbsp vinegar or lemon juice
1 tbsp xylitol
50g/2oz/½ cup mixed seeds, plus additional 1 tbsp for decoration

1 Place the buckwheat in a bowl and cover with cold water. Leave to soak overnight. Drain and rinse well.
2 Grease a 900g/2lb loaf pan and line with baking parchment.
3 Preheat the oven to 160°C/310°F/gas mark 3.
4 Place the buckwheat in a food processor with the ground sunflower seeds, flaxseed, coconut flour and chia seeds and

process to combine. Blend in the remaining ingredients until the mixture is almost smooth. Stir in the mixed seeds

5 Pour the batter into the prepared loaf pan and scatter some extra seeds on top.

6 Bake in the oven for 50 minutes until a skewer or sharp knife inserted into the loaf comes out clean.

7 Turn out onto a wire/cooling rack and leave to cool before slicing.

Bone Broth

Makes about 3l/ 105fl oz/ 12 cups

Egg Free
Nut Free
Soy Free

Bone broth can be made from any meat bones and is particularly easy using a chicken carcass. Try to use bones from an organic or grass-fed animal. Many butchers and online suppliers will sell bones or you can make use of the carcass left over from a roast. Bone broth is incredibly nourishing and ideal for supporting gut health and lowering inflammation in the body because of the collagen and glycine the bones contain. These proteins enrich the broth during the long, slow simmering. Make up a large batch and freeze in smaller containers so that you always have a handy supply of broth ready to defrost for using in soups and stews, for poaching meat or making sauces and dressings. This broth also makes a soothing hot drink. Adding a little vinegar is a useful way to draw out key minerals, such as calcium and magnesium, from the bones.

Preparation time: 10 minutes
Cooking time: 4–8 hours

1 whole organic chicken carcass, broken into pieces (ask your butcher for other chicken bits such as giblets, feet etc)
1 whole head of garlic, peeled (optional)
2 carrots, chopped
2 celery stalks, chopped
1 onion, quartered
1 bay leaf
1 tbsp black peppercorns
splash of apple cider vinegar

1 Put all the ingredients in a large flameproof casserole or saucepan with a lid. Add 3–4l/105–140fl oz/12–16 cups water to cover the bones generously, then bring to the boil

over a high heat. Reduce the heat to very low so that the stock is barely simmering. Cook for as long as possible – at least 3–4 hours but you can cook for up to about 6–8 hours. Top up with water, if needed, during cooking.

2 Strain the stock through a sieve/fine-mesh strainer. Leave to cool and store in the refrigerator for up to 5 days or freeze for up to 3 months. Once completely cooled you can skim off the fat that rises to the top.

Makes 800ml/ 28fl oz/scant 3½ cups

Coconut Yogurt

(Vegetarian)
(Vegan)
Egg Free
Soy Free

Dairy-free yogurt is easy to make at home and far cheaper than those on offer in the shops. Coconut makes wonderful yogurt, which can be thickened with agar-agar or gelatine to make it rich and creamy. Use full-fat canned coconut, ideally organic, without unnecessary fillers or sweeteners. You can use a yogurt starter kit or probiotic powder to inoculate the yogurt with beneficial bacteria but do check that the contents are dairy free. Despite its name, coconut isn't a true nut, although some people who are allergic to tree nuts (for example almonds, cashews and walnuts) may also react to coconut. As an alternative, you can make yogurt from seeds (see p.194).

Preparation time: 10 minutes
Cooking time: 2 minutes
Fermenting time: overnight or up to 24 hours

2 x 400g/14oz cans full-fat coconut milk
1 tbsp gelatine powder, or agar-agar flakes for a vegetarian/vegan option
½ tsp probiotic powder (simply open up 1–2 capsules), or a yogurt starter sachet, or 4 tbsp dairy-free yogurt

1 Heat the coconut milk and gelatine or agar-agar in a saucepan over a medium-high heat to just below boiling point. Simmer for 2 minutes and stir well, making sure the gelatine or agar-agar has dissolved. Remove from the heat and leave to cool. Stir in the probiotic powder or yogurt. For a smoother consistency pour the mixture into a blender and quickly blend.

2 Transfer to a yogurt maker or pour into a sterilized, dry vacuum flask. Leave the milk to ferment for 12–24 hours – the longer you leave it the more sour its flavour. After fermentation, stir well and put the yogurt in the refrigerator to allow the gelatine to help it set and thicken. This will take a couple of hours. Once firm you can use it in recipes or simply as it is. Store in the refrigerator for up to a week.

Nut and Seed Yogurts

Makes 625ml/ 21fl oz

Vegetarian
Vegan
Egg Free
Soy Free

Children who are allergic to nuts may be able to tolerate seeds and/ or coconut yogurt (see page 192). To make nut and seed yogurts, ideally pre-soak the nuts or seeds in water for 4 hours then drain and rinse. When making your own yogurt it is important to ensure your jar is sterilized. Any nuts can be used for this recipe and for an all-seed option try sunflower seeds.

Preparation time: 10 minutes
Fermenting time: 12 hours

125g/4oz/1 cup raw almonds, cashews or sunflower seeds, soaked then drained and rinsed
500ml/17fl oz/2 cups coconut water or water
1 tbsp sweetener (e.g maple syrup) (optional)
½ teaspoon probiotic powder (check the label to be sure it is dairy free)

1 Place all the ingredients in a powerful blender, and process until smooth and creamy. Pour into a sterilized glass jar, and set in a warm place for 9–12 hours. It should taste slightly sour.
2 Store, covered, in the refrigerator for up to a week.

Vegan Mayo

Makes about 200g/7fl oz/scant 1 cup

Vegetarian
Vegan
Egg Free
Nut Free
Soy Free

Many recipes for vegan mayonnaise are based on nuts or soy. Here is an option that is both nut and soy free. If your child is not so keen on garlic, reduce the amount. Aquafaba is the name for the viscous liquid found in a can of chickpeas/garbanzo beans. You can use this liquid as a substitute for eggs in many recipes (see page 132).

Preparation time: 5 minutes

2 garlic cloves, minced
1 tbsp fresh lemon juice
2 tsp Dijon mustard
4 tbsp aquafaba (the liquid from a can of chickpeas/garbanzo beans)
30g/1oz canned chickpeas/garbanzo beans
120ml/4fl oz/½ cup extra virgin olive oil
sea salt and freshly ground black pepper, to taste

1 Combine the garlic, lemon juice, mustard, aquafaba and chickpeas in a tall container just large enough to fit the head of a hand-held/immersion blender. Blend at high speed until completely smooth. Alternatively, blend in a food processor or blender.
2 With the blender running, slowly drizzle in the oil. A smooth, creamy emulsion should form. Add enough oil to form the consistency you like. Season with salt and pepper. Store in the refrigerator for up to 5 days.

Vegan Pesto

Makes 200g/ 7oz

Vegetarian
Vegan
Egg Free
Nut Free
Soy Free

Many children with nut allergies can react to the pine nuts traditionally used in pesto recipes; this version is made with sunflower seeds and nutritional yeast flakes instead of cheese. (You can use vegan cheese but check the labels – many brands are nut- or soy-based and may not be suitable.) For a probiotic boost you can replace the water with dairy-free yogurt or kefir.

Preparation time: 10 minutes

40g/1½oz/1 cup fresh basil (large stems removed)
40g/1½oz/1 cup fresh parsley (large stems removed)
handful of baby spinach leaves
40g/1½oz sunflower seeds
3 garlic cloves, crushed
juice of ½ lemon
3–4 tbsp nutritional yeast or vegan cheese, grated (check labels)
pinch of sea salt, to taste
3 tbsp extra virgin olive oil
3–4 tbsp water to blend

1. Put the basil, parsley, spinach, seeds, garlic, lemon juice, nutritional yeast and sea salt in a food processor or small blender and process to form a chunky paste.
2. While the machine is running, slowly add the olive oil a little at a time and scrape down the sides as needed. Then add the water a little at a time until the desired consistency is reached – a thick but pourable sauce.
3. Taste and adjust the flavour as needed, adding more nutritional yeast for a cheesier flavour or a little more salt.
4. Store, covered, in the refrigerator up to 5 days. It can also be frozen for a month.

Apple Sauerkraut

Makes 1l/35fl oz/ 4¼ cups

Vegetarian
Vegan
Egg Free
Nut Free
Soy Free

Sweet apples with spices and cabbage make this version of sauerkraut a popular fermented food for children. Try to include fermented foods daily in your child's diet to help modulate the immune system and support gut health. This sauerkraut is delicious piled on top of a baked sweet potato or homemade bread, added to salads or served alongside roast meats or fish.

Preparation time: 15 minutes
Standing time: 1 hour
Fermentation time 5–7 days

1 head of white cabbage, core removed
2 tbsp sea salt
3 red apples
1 tsp grated root ginger
½–1 tsp ground cinnamon, to taste

1. Shred the cabbage in a food processor, or chop finely with a knife. Tip into a large bowl.
2. Dissolve the sea salt in 300ml/10½ fl oz/1¼ cups warm water and stir to dissolve. Pour over the cabbage and massage the sea salt into the cabbage for about 5 minutes.
3. Cover and leave the mixture to stand for 1 hour.
4. Grate the apples or cut them into thin strips.
5. Add the apples, ginger and cinnamon to the cabbage mixture and massage in well.
6. Put the cabbage mixture with the liquid into a sterilized mason jar and pack it down until it is submerged in its own juices. Pour over additional water to ensure the mixture is fully submerged.

7. Place the lid loosely on the jar so gas can escape as fermentation takes place. Set on the work surface for 5–7 days. During fermentation the sauerkraut will bubble a little and become cloudy. Remove any scum that forms with a spoon. Taste to ensure the sauerkraut is fermented to your liking – the longer you leave it, the more sour it will become. Once opened store in the refrigerator for up to 1 month.

Breakfast

Kick start your child's day with a nourishing breakfast. Avoid shop-bought cereals and pastries which are low in nutrients, high in refined carbohydrates and sugars that will upset blood sugar levels and promote inflammation. Even if you have limited time, you will find a range of delicious ideas in this section to suit all tastes. You can also get organized and prepare many of these recipes ahead, leaving little to do in the morning. Always try and include sufficient protein and healthy fats to help stabilize blood sugar levels through the morning.

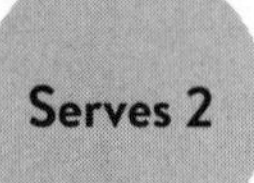

Berry Kefir Shake

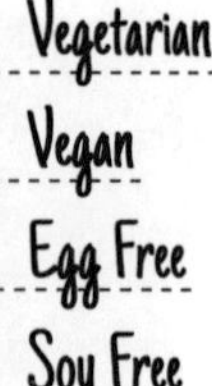

This is a delicious-tasting and nutritious breakfast drink. Smoothies are a great way to combine probiotic-rich kefir with just about any fruit. Using a combination of fresh and frozen fruit creates a thick ice-cold texture without watering down the smoothie with ice. You can also add a scoop of protein powder to the mix here, which can help to stabilize blood sugars and provide essential protein for your child's growth and development. Instead of coconut kefir you can use water kefir or some dairy-free yogurt. By including gluten-free oats and flaxseed you also provide additional fibre and healthy fats.

Preparation time: 10 minutes

- 300ml/10½ fl oz/1¼ cups coconut or water kefir (or dairy-free yogurt thinned down with a little water)
- 75g/3oz/⅔ cup strawberries or other berries
- 75g/3oz/⅔ cup frozen pitted cherries or other berries
- 2 tbsp gluten-free rolled oats or quinoa flakes or buckwheat flakes
- 1 tbsp ground flaxseed (optional)

Simply place all the ingredients in a food processor and blend until smooth and creamy.

Carrot Cake Granola

Makes 12 servings

Vegetarian
Vegan
Egg Free
(Nut Free)
Soy Free

A fabulous granola with the flavours of carrot cake! This is a great way to use up any carrot pulp left over from juicing. Orange juice and xylitol sweeten this gluten-free granola without the need for sugars or syrups. It's delicious served with dairy-free yogurt and fruit as a healthy breakfast or snack. You can make this nut free by omitting the coconut and using olive oil rather than coconut oil. Make up a batch of this granola and store in an airtight container for up to 2 weeks.

Preparation time: 15 minutes
Cooking time: 30 minutes

60g/2½oz coconut oil, softened (or 60ml/2½ fl oz olive oil for a nut-free option)
zest and juice of 1 orange
2 tbsp xylitol
1 tsp vanilla extract
60g/2½oz carrot, grated, or leftover carrot pulp
2 tsp ground cinnamon
100g/3½oz/1 cup mixed seeds (sunflower, sesame and pumpkin)
350g/12oz/3½ cups gluten-free rolled oats, quinoa flakes, millet flakes, rice flakes or buckwheat flakes (or a mixture)
60g/2½oz/⅔ cup unsweetened desiccated/dried shredded coconut or coconut flakes (omit for a nut-free option)
60g/2½oz/½ cup goji berries, dried berries or raisins

1 Preheat the oven to 180°C/350°F/gas mark 4 and lightly grease a baking sheet.

2 Put the oil, orange zest and juice, xylitol, vanilla and carrot in a blender or food processor and blend to form a thick paste.
3 Put the remaining ingredients except the dried fruit in a large bowl and stir the mixture. Pour over the orange paste and use your hands to massage everything together so that all the dry ingredients are coated.
4 Spread out the granola in a thin layer on the baking sheet.
5 Cook for 30 minutes until lightly golden, stirring occasionally during cooking to prevent burning.
6 Leave the granola to cool then stir in the dried fruit. Store in an airtight container.

American Pancakes with Berry Compôte

Makes 8 pancakes

Vegetarian
(Egg Free)
(Nut Free)
(Soy Free)

Children adore pancakes and these light and fluffy American-style ones are a healthy treat served with the berry sauce. Buckwheat flour adds a lovely rich, nutty flavour and provides plenty of fibre to support gut health. It is also rich in key minerals, including manganese, copper and magnesium that help to boost energy levels. It also provides quercetin, an antioxidant known for its antihistamine properties. You can make this egg free by using commercial egg replacer. Alternatively, mix 1 tbsp potato flour with ¼ tsp xanthum gum and 2 tbsp water or mash up ½ banana and add to the batter to replace the egg.

Preparation time: 15 minutes
Cooking time: 25 minutes

50g/2oz/½ cup buckwheat flour or gluten-free plain/all-purpose flour (or see page 182)
75g/3oz/¾ cup gluten-free plain/all-purpose flour (or see page 182)
2 tsp gluten-free baking powder
pinch of sea salt
2 tbsp xylitol, erythritol or stevia, to taste
100ml/3½fl oz/scant ½ cup dairy-free milk
60ml/2½fl oz dairy-free yogurt or coconut kefir (or dairy-free milk)
1 egg, beaten, or egg replacer (see page 132)
2 tbsp melted dairy-free spread, coconut oil or olive oil
olive oil or coconut oil, for frying

Berry compôte

200g/7oz mixed berries, fresh or frozen
2 tbsp water
1 tsp xylitol, to taste (optional)
2 tsp cornflour/cornstarch
dairy-free yogurt, to serve (optional)

1 First make the compôte. Put the berries, water and xylitol in a pan, cover and simmer gently over a low heat for 2–3 minutes to soften. Add a little extra water if needed. Mix together the cornflour/cornstarch with 2 tbsp water to form a smooth paste. Add to the pan and stir for 1–2 minutes until the mixture thickens. Set aside. This can be made ahead of time and kept in the refrigerator until required.
2 For the pancakes, gently sift the flours, baking powder, salt and xylitol into a bowl.
3 In a separate bowl, whisk together the milk, yogurt, egg (or egg-free alternative) and melted spread or oil.
4 Pour the milk mixture into the flour mixture and beat with a wire whisk to create a smooth batter. Leave it to stand for a few minutes. Alternatively simply place all the ingredients in a blender and process until smooth.
5 Heat a non-stick frying pan over a medium heat and add a little coconut oil or olive oil.
6 When the pan is hot add a ladle of batter (or more if your frying pan is big enough to cook several pancakes at once). Cook until bubbles show on the top of the pancake then flip it over and cook on the other side until golden.
7 Repeat, adding extra oil as needed, until you have used all the batter.
8 Serve the pancakes with the compôte and dairy-free yogurt if wished.

Apple Streusel Muffins

Makes 10 muffins

These tasty little muffins are perfect for breakfast or packed lunches. Your child will also love these warm from the oven for an after-school snack. Apples are a good source of several antioxidants, including quercetin, catechins, and chlorogenic acid, all known for their anti-inflammatory properties. The polyphenols present in apples also support the growth of friendly gut bacteria, which play a key role in our immune health. For a change, use seeds or dairy-free chocolate chunks in place of the dried apple.

Vegetarian
Vegan
Egg Free
(Nut Free)
(Soy Free)

Preparation time: 15 minutes
Cooking time: 25 minutes

225g gluten-free flour blend (see page 182)
pinch of sea salt
1 tbsp gluten-free baking powder
40g/1½oz/scant ⅓ cup xylitol
1 tbsp ground flaxseed
4 tbsp olive oil, melted coconut oil or dairy-free spread
2 red apples, grated
160ml/5½fl oz/scant ¾ cup dairy-free milk
1 tsp ground cinnamon
50g/2oz/½ cup dried apple pieces, diced (optional)

Topping
1 tbsp xylitol
30g/1oz gluten-free rolled oats
¼ tsp ground cinnamon
1 tbsp olive oil

1. Grease and line a muffin pan with muffin cases/liners.
2. Preheat the oven to 190°C/375°F/gas mark 5.

3. Place the flour, salt, baking powder and xylitol in a food processor or large bowl and mix together.
4. Add the remaining ingredients and mix well. Fold in the apple pieces if using.
5. To make the streusel topping simply mix all the ingredients together in a small bowl.
6. Spoon the batter into the cases and top with a little of the topping.
7. Bake in the oven for 20–25 minutes or until firm to touch and golden.
8. Transfer to a wire/cooling rack and leave to cool.

Fruity Millet Porridge

Serves 6

Vegetarian
Vegan
Egg Free
(Nut Free)
(Soy Free)

If your child is not able to tolerate gluten-free rolled oats here is a delicious alternative. This creamy porridge uses whole millet grain to provide plenty of fibre, which can help balance blood sugars for sustained energy. You can make this the night before and heat it in the morning to save time. For a nut-free option replace the coconut cream with soy cream or use extra dairy-free milk.

Preparation time: 10 minutes
Cooking time: 30 minutes

150g/5oz/¾ cup millet grain
750ml/26fl oz/3¼ cups water
2 ripe pears, peeled, cored and diced
150ml/5fl oz/⅔ cup dairy-free milk
100ml/3½fl oz/scant ½ cup coconut cream, soy cream or additional dairy free milk
8 dried apricots
1 tsp ground cinnamon
1 tbsp ground flaxseed

1. Put the millet and water in a saucepan and bring to the boil. Simmer, covered, for 15 minutes. Add the pear and continue to cook for a further 15 minutes until all the water has been absorbed. Set aside.
2. Put the remaining ingredients in a blender or food processor and process until smooth.
3. Pour the coconut cream mixture into the millet and mix well. Serve hot or cold.

Breakfast Seed Bars

Makes 16 bars

Vegetarian
Vegan
Egg Free
(Nut Free)
(Soy Free)

These bars are perfect for a 'grab and go' breakfast option and are ideal for snacks and packed lunches, too. If your child is allergic to coconut you can use 140g (5oz) of tahini (sesame seed paste) or other seed butter instead of the coconut milk and skip step 2. These bars are far healthier than shop-bought cereal bars.

Preparation time: 15 minutes
Cooking time: 45 minutes

1 x 400g/14oz can full-fat coconut milk
75g/3oz/scant ¾ cup xylitol
120g/4oz coconut oil or cacao butter or dairy-free spread
pinch of sea salt
1 tsp ground cinnamon
200g/7oz/2 cups gluten-free rolled oats, millet, buckwheat or rice flakes
60g/2½ oz/1 cup rice puffs
30g/1oz dried cranberries
30g/1oz pumpkin seeds
1 tbsp chia seeds

1 Preheat the oven to 180°C/350°F/gas mark 4.
2 Put the coconut milk into a small saucepan and add the xylitol. Stir over a gentle heat until the xylitol has dissolved. Bring to a boil and simmer for 20 minutes until thickened.
3 Add the coconut oil or dairy-free spread and melt gently. Allow to cool slightly before using.
4 Put all the remaining ingredients into a large bowl. Pour over the coconut mixture and stir well to combine.
5 Grease and line a 20cm/8in square traybake pan. Press the mixture firmly into the pan. Bake in the oven for 25 minutes until golden. Cool completely in the pan before slicing.

Breakfast Bean Burritos

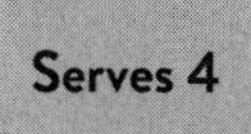

Easy to make and assemble, these burritos are a delicious breakfast option that are also perfect as a lunch or evening meal. Beans, onions and garlic are all prebiotics which mean they help support the growth of beneficial bacteria in our gut and in turn help support a healthy immune system.

Vegetarian
Vegan
Egg Free
Soy Free

Preparation time: 15 minutes
Cooking time: 15 minutes

1 tbsp olive oil
1 onion, finely chopped
1 red pepper, diced
1 garlic clove, crushed
1 x 400g/14oz can plum tomatoes
1 x 400g/14oz can red kidney beans, drained
2 tsp tomato purée/paste
½ tsp chilli powder

To serve

4 corn tortillas (see page 184) or gluten-free tortillas
Creamy guacamole (see page 283)

1 Heat the oil in a frying pan and sauté the onion, pepper and garlic for 5 minutes until the onion is soft. Tip in the tomatoes and kidney beans, add the tomato purée/paste and chilli powder and simmer for 10 minutes until the sauce has reduced. Use a potato masher to crush the beans and tomatoes slightly.
2 Microwave the tortillas for 10 seconds to soften. To serve, top a tortilla with beans and guacamole and roll it up. Repeat with the remaining tortillas.

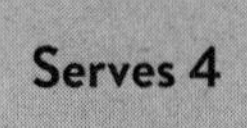

Breakfast Sweet Potato Chorizo Hash

Egg Free
Nut Free
Soy Free

Sweet potato is naturally rich in betacarotene, which the body converts to vitamin A, one of the most important vitamins for the immune system and gut health. You can swap the butter/lima beans for any canned beans you have available, and gluten-free sausages make a good alternative to the chorizo. Read the labels carefully as some chorizo can contain dairy.

Preparation time: 15 minutes
Cooking time: 25 minutes

1 sweet potato (about 300g/10½oz), peeled and cut into 2cm chunks
1 tbsp olive oil
200g/7oz cooking chorizo sausages, skinned and crumbled or finely chopped
1 red onion, diced
1 x 400g/14oz can butter/lima beans, drained and rinsed
1 red chilli, deseeded and diced
handful of parsley, chopped, to serve

1. Boil the sweet potatoes for 5 minutes until just soft, then drain and put back in the pan to steam dry.
2. Meanwhile, heat the oil in a large frying pan and cook the chorizo and onion for 5 minutes until softened. Add the sweet potatoes, butter/lima beans and chilli and cook for 20 minutes or until the potatoes are golden and crispy. Press the potato mixture down slightly to brown.
3. Sprinkle over the parsley to serve.

Baked Beans on Waffles

(Egg Free)
(Nut Free)
(Soy Free)

Baked beans are always a hit with children but shop-bought brands are often high in sugar and salt. These are easy to make and much healthier. You can make up a batch the day before. These waffles can also be made sweet by adding 1 tbsp of xylitol to the batter and serving them topped with fruit and dairy-free yogurt. For an egg-free version, mix together 2 tbsp potato flour or tapioca starch, ½ tsp xanthum gum, 1 tbsp olive oil and 4 tbsp water. For a sweet egg-free option replace the eggs with 1 ripe banana and add ½ tsp xanthum gum and a little extra dairy-free milk if the batter is too thick.

Preparation time: 15 minutes
Cooking time: 16 minutes

Baked Beans

1 tbsp olive oil
2 garlic cloves, crushed
¼–½ tsp smoked paprika
300g/10½oz passata
1 tbsp tomato purée/paste
1 x 400g/14oz can haricot/navy beans, drained
¼ tsp stevia (optional)
1 tsp apple cider vinegar (optional)

Waffles

2 tbsp olive oil
250ml/9fl oz/1 cup dairy-free milk
1 tsp apple cider vinegar or lemon juice
2 eggs
250g/9oz/2¼ cups gluten-free flour blend (see page 182) or brown rice flour
1 tsp gluten-free baking powder
1 tbsp ground flaxseed

1. To make the beans heat the oil in saucepan over a medium heat. Add the garlic and sauté for 1 minute. Add the smoked paprika, passata and tomato purée/paste and simmer for 10 minutes until the sauce has thickened. Tip in the beans and simmer for a further 5 minutes. If your children like their beans slightly tangy add the stevia and vinegar and stir.
2. Meanwhile make the waffles. Simply place all the ingredients in a blender or use a stick blender and blend until smooth. It should form a thick batter. Heat and grease your waffle iron. Pour in a quarter of the batter and cook according to the manufacturer's instructions. Repeat with the remaining batter.
3. Serve the waffles topped with a spoonful of baked beans.

Salmon Kedgeree

If you have leftover rice you can assemble this dish in minutes. Oily fish such as salmon is rich in omega-3 fats which are not only essential for brain health but can help to lower inflammation, making them useful for reducing allergy symptoms. The eggs are optional – omit them if your child has an egg allergy.

(Egg Free)
Nut Free
Soy Free

Preparation time: 15 minutes
Cooking time: 25 minutes

200g/7oz/1 cup basmati rice
500ml/17fl oz/2 cups water
2 eggs (optional)
400g/14oz hot-smoked salmon or trout fillets
2 tbsp olive oil
1 red onion, chopped
2 tsp mild curry paste (check labels) or use 1 tbsp curry powder
150g/5oz/1 cup frozen peas
2 tomatoes, deseeded and diced
sea salt and freshly ground black pepper
handful of parsley, roughly chopped
Juice of ½ lemon

1. Place the rice in a pan and cover with the water. Bring to the boil then put the lid on the pan and simmer over a very low heat for 20 minutes. Turn off the heat and leave the rice to stand for 5 minutes.
2. Meanwhile, if you are including the eggs, place a small pan of water over a high heat and bring to a rolling boil. Carefully add the eggs and boil for 6 minutes. Drain and cool immediately under cold running water.

3. Flake the fish and set aside.
4. Heat the oil in a large frying pan or saucepan. Fry the onion over a low heat until soft, then add the curry paste and cook for 1–2 minutes. Add the cooked rice, peas, tomatoes and fish. Season well. Stir over a moderate heat for about 5 minutes until hot, then stir in the parsley and lemon juice.
5. Shell the eggs, if using, quarter and arrange on top of the kedgeree to serve.

Lunches / light dishes

Keep your child focused and alert all afternoon with a nutritious, satisfying lunch. Whether you are looking for packed-lunch ideas beyond the humble sandwich or family friendly lunches for the weekend, in this chapter you will find a whole range of delicious and nourishing dishes to enjoy. Designed with busy parents in mind, many of these recipes can be prepared in advance. The focus is on nutrient-rich ingredients designed to support a healthy immune system and gut health and lower inflammation. By providing a nourishing lunch for your child you will boost their energy levels, helping them to make the most of their day.

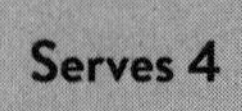

Roasted Red Pepper Tortilla Soup

Vegetarian
Vegan
Egg Free
Nut Free
Soy Free

This warming, hearty vegan soup is simple to prepare and packed with antioxidant-rich vegetables. Plant antioxidants – particularly quercetin and anthocyanins – are particularly beneficial to any child with allergies because they help to lower the activity of mast cells, which release histamine during allergic reactions. Kidney beans provide plenty of fibre and protein to keep blood sugar levels balanced and energy levels high.

Preparation time: 10 minutes
Cooking time: 22 minutes

1 tbsp olive oil
1 red onion, diced
1 garlic clove, crushed
1 celery stalk, diced
2 carrots, chopped
1 tsp taco seasoning (check labels)
½ tsp ground cumin
600ml/20fl oz/2½ cups vegetable stock
2 tomatoes, chopped
250g/9oz roasted red peppers from a jar, drained and chopped
sea salt and freshly ground black pepper, to taste
100g/3½oz canned sweetcorn/corn kernels, drained
100g/3½oz canned kidney beans, drained and rinsed
60g/2½oz corn tortilla chips (check labels), plus a few extra to serve

1 Heat the olive oil in a large pan. Gently sauté the onion, garlic, celery and carrots for 5 minutes until the onion has softened. Add the spices and stir to coat.
2 Add the stock, tomatoes and peppers and bring to a boil. Cover and simmer for 15 minutes until the vegetables are tender. Season to taste.
3 Pour the mixture into a blender and process until smooth. Add the sweetcorn/corn kernels, kidney beans and tortilla chips and pulse briefly to chop up the ingredients slightly.
4 Pour the soup back into the pan and warm through. Spoon into bowls and top with a few tortilla chips.

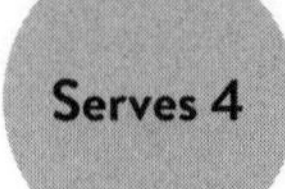

Chicken Noodle Soup

Egg Free
Nut Free
Soy Free

This meal in a bowl is wonderfully nourishing, and particularly good for immune health. Homemade bone broth (see page 190) is rich in collagen and glycine, known for their gut-healing properties. Ginger and turmeric are gently warming spices that add more than flavour; they are good decongestants, and have anti-inflammatory and antihistamine properties. If you already have cooked chicken left over, then use this to save time.

Preparation time: 15 minutes
Cooking time: 18 minutes

- 2 chicken breasts (or 200g/7oz leftover cooked chicken)
- 400ml/14fl oz/1⅔ cups chicken stock or homemade bone broth (see page 190)
- 1 tsp fish sauce
- 1 tsp rice wine vinegar
- 200g/7oz rice noodles
- 1 tbsp olive oil
- 4 spring onions/scallions, sliced
- 2 celery stalks, diced
- 2 carrots, diced
- ½ red chilli, deseeded and diced
- 2 garlic cloves, crushed
- ½ tsp grated root ginger
- ¼ tsp ground turmeric
- 1 x 400g/14oz can chopped tomatoes
- 4 button mushrooms, sliced
- 100g/3½oz baby spinach leaves
- sea salt and freshly ground black pepper, to taste
- handful of coriander/cilantro leaves, chopped, to serve

1 Place the chicken breast in a pan and pour over the stock and add the fish sauce and vinegar. Bring to the boil and simmer for 15 minutes. Turn off the heat and leave the chicken to continue to cook in the stock for a further 5 minutes. Remove

the chicken from the stock and set aside, reserving the stock. When cool enough to handle, shred the meat.

2 Meanwhile cook the noodles according to the package directions, drain and rinse.

3 Heat the olive oil in a large pan and sauté the spring onions/scallions, celery, carrots, chilli, garlic, ginger and turmeric for 3–5 minutes until the celery is soft. Pour over the reserved chicken stock and add the chopped tomatoes and mushrooms. Cook gently for 10 minutes until the vegetables are soft. Add the shredded chicken, spinach and drained noodles. Heat through for 2–3 minutes. Taste, and season with salt and pepper if needed.

4 Spoon into bowls and top with chopped coriander/cilantro leaves.

Rice Paper Rolls

Makes 8 rolls

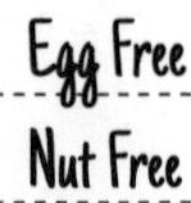

Rice paper rolls are an ideal allergy-free finger food for children because you can vary the filling ingredients according to your child's tastes and allergies. Prawns/shrimp are a good source of omega-3 fatty acids and contain astaxanthin, another antioxidant known for its anti-inflammatory benefits.

Preparation time: 15 minutes

1 small carrot
½ cucumber
100g/3½oz soft lettuce, shredded
125g/4oz cooked prawns/shrimp, roughly chopped
handful of mint leaves, chopped
sea salt and freshly ground black pepper, to taste
8 rice paper sheets

Dipping sauce

1 tbsp xylitol
2 tbsp lime juice
1 tbsp fish sauce
1 tbsp tamari (gluten-free soy sauce)
1 garlic clove, crushed
pinch of chilli flakes (optional)

1. Prepare the dipping sauce by mixing all the ingredients together in a small bowl.
2. Use a swivel-head vegetable peeler to slice the cucumber and carrot into ribbons. Place all the remaining filling ingredients in a bowl and mix well. Season to taste.

3 Place one sheet of rice paper in a shallow bowl of warm water until just softened. Carefully transfer the sheet from the water onto a dish-towel covered board.
4 Place a little of the carrot and cucumber in the middle of the sheet. Top with some of the remaining filling ingredients. Fold the corner point nearest to you up and over the filling, folding in the sides after the first complete turn of the roll. Repeat with the remaining rice paper sheets and filling ingredients.
5 Serve with the dipping sauce.

Makes 16/ serves 4–6

Falafel Bites with Salsa and Minted Dip

Vegetarian
Vegan
Egg Free
(Nut Free)
Soy Free

These little nuggets make a tasty packed-lunch filler as an alternative to sandwiches. Serve them in Little Gem lettuce leaves with a fruity salsa and probiotic-rich dip for a light and healthy option. Chickpeas/garbanzo beans are a great vegetarian protein option and a source of energizing B vitamins, magnesium and iron.

Preparation time: 20 minutes
Cooking time: 20 minutes

1 x 400g/14oz can chickpeas/ garbanzo beans, drained and rinsed
3 garlic cloves, crushed
1 small red onion, finely chopped
handful of coriander/cilantro leaves, chopped
handful of parsley, chopped
1 tbsp ground flaxseed
½ tsp ground cumin
1 tbsp olive oil
sea salt and freshly ground black pepper
150g/5oz/1¼ cups stale gluten-free breadcrumbs (or dry out fresh crumbs in a cool oven for a few minutes)

2 Little Gem lettuces, leaves separated, to serve

Minted Dip

⅓ cucumber
150g/5oz/⅔ cup homemade dairy-free yogurt (see page 194) or other dairy free yogurt
1 tsp lemon juice
handful of fresh mint leaves, chopped

Fruity Salsa

8 cherry tomatoes
1 spring onion/scallion, finely chopped
½ cucumber, deseeded and diced
½ mango, peeled and diced
30g/1oz canned sweetcorn/corn kernels, drained
squeeze of lemon juice
salt and pepper, to taste

1 Preheat the oven to 200°C/400°F/gas mark 6. Grease a baking sheet with oil.
2 Put the chickpeas/garbanzo beans in a food processor and process to break them up. Add the garlic, onion, herbs, flaxseed, cumin, olive oil and half of the breadcrumbs and process until you have a fairly smooth purée. Season to taste.
3 Spread out the remaining breadcrumbs on a plate.
4 Form the mixture into about 12 walnut-size balls, then roll them lightly in the remaining breadcrumbs. Place them on the greased baking sheet, then bake in the oven for about 20 minutes or until golden, turning once.
5 To make the dip, coarsely grate the cucumber and squeeze in a clean dish towel to remove excess water. Mix all the ingredients together in a small bowl.
6 For the salsa simply mix all the ingredients together.
7 To serve, place a falafel in a Little Gem lettuce leaf and top with some of the dip and salsa.

Homemade Pasties

Serves 4

(Egg Free)
Nut Free
(Soy Free)

Pasties are another great option for lunch boxes and meals on the go. It's easy enough to vary the size of the pasties depending on the age of your child. Red meats like beef as well as carrots provide a valuable source of glutamine, an amino acid that plays a key role in maintaining a healthy gut lining and healing a leaky gut. You can make these vegetarian by swapping the beef for a can of kidney beans.

Preparation time: 20 minutes
Cooking time: 35 minutes

1 tbsp olive oil
300g/10½oz minced/ground beef
1 onion
1 sweet potato
2 carrots
1 tbsp tamari (gluten-free soy sauce) (optional)
3 tbsp passata or homemade tomato ketchup (see page 255)

1 quantity of shortcrust pastry/pie dough (see page 183)

Beaten egg, to glaze (or water/non-dairy milk for egg-free option)

1 Heat the oil in a frying pan or casserole dish. Fry the beef, stirring frequently, until it is no longer pink.
2 Grate the onion, sweet potato and carrots and add to the pan with the tamari, if using, and passata or tomato ketchup. Cover and simmer for 15 minutes or until the beef is completely cooked through. Leave to cool before using.

3. Roll out the pastry dough between two sheets of cling film/ plastic wrap. Using a bowl or plate about 15cm/6in diameter as a guide, cut out four rounds.
4. Place a quarter of the mixture in the middle of each round. Brush the edges of the pastry dough with beaten egg. Bring up the edges of the dough and crimp the edges together to seal. Transfer to a baking sheet and brush with the beaten egg, non-dairy milk or water. Bake in the oven for 20 minutes until golden brown.

Pineapple & Pork Salad

Serves 4

Egg Free
Nut Free
Soy Free

Pineapple and pork come together to make a fruity, protein-packed salad. Pineapple contains plenty of vitamins and minerals as well as an enzyme called bromelain, which is known for its powerful anti-inflammatory properties.

Preparation time: 15 minutes
Cooking time: 10 minutes

1 tbsp olive oil
250g/9oz minced/ground pork
200g/7oz fresh pineapple chunks (or from a can in juice, drained)
4 spring onions/scallions, thinly sliced
1 red pepper, deseeded and diced
½ cucumber, halved lengthways then sliced
2 Little Gem lettuces, shredded
handful of mint leaves, chopped
handful of basil leaves, chopped

Dressing

juice of 3 limes
2 tsp xylitol
1 garlic clove, crushed
2 tbsp fish sauce

1 To make the dressing, put all the ingredients in a jar, screw on the lid tightly and shake vigorously to combine.
2 Heat the oil in a sauté pan and add the pork. Cook for 8–10 minutes until browned and cooked through, breaking up the meat with a wooden spoon. Cool slightly then place in a large bowl with the remaining ingredients.
3 To serve, pour the dressing over the salad, mix gently and spoon onto plates.

Pizza

Makes 1 large pizza/ Serves 6

This makes a delicious gluten-free pizza. The addition of olive oil keeps the base lovely and moist. This is a great recipe for getting the children involved in cooking and choosing their toppings. Tomatoes are rich in lycopene, an antioxidant that helps to balance the immune system, and decrease the allergic response and inflammation of cells in the lungs, making it particularly beneficial for asthma.

Vegetarian
Vegan
Egg Free
Nut Free
Soy Free*

* for the base; choose toppings that suit your child's allergy needs

Preparation time: 15 minutes
Cooking time: 23 minutes
Proving time: 45 minutes

2 tsp caster/superfine sugar
200ml/7fl oz/scant 1 cup lukewarm water
2 x 7g sachets fast-action/instant active dried yeast
300g/10½oz/2⅔ cups gluten-free bread flour blend (see page 182), plus extra for dusting
1 tsp xanthan gum
1 tsp gluten-free baking powder
½ tsp bicarbonate of soda/baking soda
1 tsp sea salt
2 tbsp olive oil
1 tsp apple cider vinegar

Topping

3 tbsp passata plus sliced cherry tomatoes, wafer ham, sweetcorn/corn kernels, red pepper, sliced mushrooms, dairy-free cheese, as wished
fresh basil leaves, to serve

1 To make the dough, mix together the sugar, warm water and yeast. Leave in a warm place for 5–10 minutes or until it starts to froth and bubble.
2 Place the remaining dry ingredients in a large mixing bowl. Add the yeast mixture, olive oil and vinegar and beat together to form a soft, wet dough. Cover with cling film/plastic wrap and leave to prove for 45 minutes.
3 Preheat the oven to 200°C/400°F/gas mark 6.
4 Place the dough on a lightly greased baking sheet or pizza sheet. Flour your hands and flatten out the dough (or use a rolling pin) to form a circle about 20cm/8in in diameter.
5 Bake the base for 8 minutes and then remove from the oven. Spread the passata over the base and arrange your chosen toppings. Bake for a further 10–15 minutes until cooked.
6 Top with fresh basil leaves and serve immediately. Any leftovers make an ideal packed-lunch option for the following day.

Mexican Taco Chicken Salad

Serves 4

Egg Free
Nut Free
Soy Free

This crunchy chicken salad is fresh, healthy and packed with colourful vegetables. Avocados provide plenty of monounsaturated oleic acid, a healthy fat known for its anti-inflammatory benefits. Studies have also shown that eating avocado with veggies can dramatically increase the amount of antioxidants you take in. Try this for variety in your child's lunchbox.

Preparation time: 15 minutes

2 Little Gem lettuces, shredded
100g/3½oz canned sweetcorn/corn kernels, drained
12 cherry tomatoes, halved
handful of pitted olives, halved
⅓ cucumber, halved lengthways, deseeded and cut into slices
2 cooked chicken breasts, shredded
½ avocado, pitted and diced
60g/2½oz corn tortilla chips (check labels)

Dressing

½ avocado, pitted
1 garlic clove, crushed
1 tbsp lemon juice
1 tbsp olive oil
sea salt and freshly ground black pepper

1 Make the dressing by putting all the ingredients in a blender with 1–2 tbsp water. Process to form a thick, smooth dressing.
2 Put the lettuce, sweetcorn/corn kernels, tomatoes, olives, cucumber and chicken in a bowl, along with the remaining half of the avocado. Drizzle over the avocado dressing and scatter with the tortilla chips to serve.

Sandwich Fillers

If you are making up a lunch box for a child with allergies, you'll want plenty of ideas to keep their midday meal varied throughout the week. Here are some healthy options for sandwich or wrap fillers to try.

Non-vegetarian/vegan filling options for sandwiches and wraps

Salmon and cucumber: Drain and mash a can of boneless salmon. For a creamy taste stir in a spoonful of homemade mayo (see recipe opposite) or dairy-free yogurt (see page 194). Deseed and dice ⅓ cucumber and mix in with the salmon.

Chicken and Apple: Top bread with shredded chicken and thin slices of apple (drizzle a little lemon juice over the apple slices to stop them browning).

Refried Beans: Dice ½ onion and sauté in a little oil until soft. Add a can of drained, rinsed kidney beans, 1 tbsp tomato purée/paste and a little smoked paprika and ground cumin to taste. Mash lightly to create a chunky texture.

Carrot and Raisin: Mix together a grated carrot, a handful of raisins and a spoonful of homemade mayo (see page 195), dairy-free yogurt (see page 194) or hummus.

Steak and Guacamole: Spread guacamole on bread and top with thinly sliced cooked steak.

Chicken with Fruity Coleslaw: Use the apple sauerkraut (see page 196) and mix in a little homemade mayo (see page 195) or dairy-free yogurt (see page 194) to make a healthy coleslaw. Use to top shredded cooked chicken breast.

Roast Beef and Sauerkraut: Top slices of beef with homemade sauerkraut (see page 197)

Salmon, Tomato and Alfalfa: Drain a can of boneless salmon and mash with a little tomato ketchup (see page 255). Spread on bread and top with alfalfa sprouts or cress.

Creamy Smoked Mackerel: Skin and flake smoked mackerel fillets then mix with a little homemade mayo (see page 195), or dairy-free yogurt (see page 194).

BLT: Use slices of prosciutto, slices of tomato, avocado and Little Gem lettuce leaves.

Chicken Pesto: Mix 1–2 tbsp homemade pesto (see page 195) with 3 tbsp homemade mayonnaise (see page 195) then toss in shredded cooked chicken breast. Spread on bread and top with lettuce or baby spinach.

Cucumber and Prawns/shrimp: Make the minted dip (see page 222), and mix in baby cooked prawns/shrimp.

Mains

Finding family dishes that everyone will enjoy can be tricky at the best of times, and particularly if you are catering for various allergies. The recipes in this section are designed to be enjoyed by the whole family, avoiding the need to cook separate allergy-free options. The focus, as with all recipes in this book, is on nourishing recipes that help to address immune imbalances, calm inflammation and support gut health. To save time, many of the recipes can be prepared ahead or left to slow cook in the oven with minimum fuss.

Slow-cooked Beef Chilli

Serves 4

Egg Free
Nut Free
Soy Free

Beef chilli, served with cornbread (see page 236) or rice, is a hearty gluten-free dish to serve your children and the great thing about this recipe is you can throw it all together in minutes and then leave it to cook slowly in the oven. The addition of liver provides plenty of vitamins A and D, both essential for healthy immune function as well as to support gut healing. Remember to check labels of stock cubes to ensure they are free from gluten and dairy.

Preparation time: 15 minutes
Cooking time: 1 hour 40 minutes

2 tbsp olive oil
450g/1lb minced/ground beef
150g/5oz chicken livers, finely diced
4 streaky bacon slices, chopped
1 red onion, finely chopped
2 garlic cloves, crushed
2 tbsp smoked paprika
½ tsp chilli powder
1 tsp ground cumin
2 tbsp tomato purée/paste
2 tbsp unsweetened cocoa powder
600g/1lb 4oz passata
1 x 400g/14oz can red kidney beans, drained and rinsed
1 x 400g/14oz can chopped tomatoes
1 red pepper, deseeded and diced
2 beef stock cubes, crumbled (check labels)
sea salt and freshly ground black pepper, to taste
cornbread, (see page 236), to serve

1. Preheat the oven to 150°C/300°F/gas mark 2.
2. Heat the olive oil in a large ovenproof casserole dish and brown the beef, livers and bacon for 5 minutes.
3. Add the onion, garlic and spices and cook for 5 minutes, stirring to prevent it sticking.
4. Add the tomato purée/paste, cocoa powder, passata, kidney beans, chopped tomatoes, red pepper and stock cubes to the pan and stir well to combine. Season with salt and pepper.
5. Transfer the dish to the oven, cover and cook for 1½ hours. Check occasionally and add a little water if needed. Serve with cornbread.

Cornbread

Makes 12 slices

Vegetarian
(Nut Free)
(Soy Free)

This is a great bread to serve with beef chilli (see page 234). It is also delicious cut into chunks and served with soup. The addition of apple keeps this bread wonderfully moist.

Preparation time: 15 minutes
Cooking time: 35 minutes

150g/5oz/1 cup fine polenta/ yellow cornmeal
150g gluten-free bread flour (see page 182)
2 tsp gluten-free baking powder
1 tsp bicarbonate of soda/baking soda
1 tsp sea salt
2 eggs
2 tbsp olive oil
1 tbsp maple syrup or xylitol (optional)
200ml/7fl oz/scant 1 cup dairy-free milk
125g/4oz apple purée

1. Preheat the oven to 180°C/350°F/gas mark 4. Grease and line a 20cm/8in square or round baking pan.
2. Sift the polenta/cornmeal, flour, baking powder and bicarbonate of soda/baking soda into a large bowl and stir in the salt. In a separate bowl, beat together the eggs, oil, syrup or xylitol if using, milk and apple purée. Pour into the flour mixture and combine to create a soft batter.
3. Pour the batter into the prepared pan and bake in the oven for 35 minutes, until risen and golden. To check the cornbread is cooked through, insert a skewer into the middle of the loaf; it should come out clean. Leave to cool in the pan for a few minutes then turn out and cut into bars. Serve warm or cold.

Chow Mein

Serves 4

Egg Free

Nut Free

My version of this Chinese classic is made with beefsteak but it is equally delicious with minced/ground beef, with chicken or, for a vegetarian-protein option, you could use a couple of cans of beans of your choice. Chinese/Napa cabbage contains large amounts of carotenoids and vitamin C, which are known to help reduce allergy symptoms by lowering histamine. As always, check labels carefully: not all oyster sauces are gluten free. If you want to avoid oyster sauce altogether because your child has fish allergies, simply replace it with extra tamari.

Preparation time: 15 minutes
Marinating time: 20 minutes
Cooking time: 15 minutes

2 tbsp tamari (gluten-free soy sauce)
2 tbsp Chinese rice wine or dry sherry
2 tbsp gluten-free oyster sauce (check labels)
½ tsp toasted sesame oil (optional)
2 tsp cornflour/cornstarch
300g/10½oz sirloin steak, trimmed and cut into strips
250g/9oz rice noodles
4 tbsp olive oil or coconut oil
50ml/2fl oz chicken stock
1 tsp grated root ginger
2 garlic cloves, crushed
3 spring onions/scallions, finely chopped
100g/3½oz button mushrooms, thinly sliced
½ small Chinese/Napa cabbage, shredded
100g/3½ oz mangetout/snowpeas
100g/3½ oz bean sprouts

1 Mix together in a medium bowl half the soy sauce, rice wine and oyster sauce (1 tbsp of each) with the sesame oil and half (1 tsp) the cornflour/cornstarch. Add the steak, toss to coat, and leave to marinate for 20 minutes.
2 Cook the noodles in boiling water for just 30 seconds. Drain and toss in 1 tbsp olive oil.
3 Mix together the remaining sauces, rice wine and cornflour/cornstarch and stir in the stock.
4 Heat 2 tbsp olive oil in a wok or large frying pan. Add the noodles and cook for 5–7 minutes until the underside is golden. Flip over the noodle 'cake' and cook for about 3 minutes, until lightly golden. Place on a warm serving plate.
5 Add the remaining oil to the wok and, when hot, add the steak. Stir-fry for 2–3 minutes, then tip out onto a plate.
6 Add the ginger, garlic and spring onions/scallions; after 30 seconds, add the mushrooms. Cook for 2 minutes, then add the remaining ingredients, stir-frying until the cabbage has wilted. Pour in the reserved sauce mixture, return the steak and bring to the boil. Stir well and, once bubbling, serve over the noodles.

Fruity Lamb Tagine

Serves 6

Egg Free
Nut Free
Soy Free

This is another family dish that can be prepared ahead and left to cook in the oven. Tagines are perfect for sneaking in plenty of vegetables, too. Lamb is a great source of bioavailable iron, zinc, B vitamins and selenium, all nutrients to support immune health, growth and development and maintain energy levels. For a vegetarian option you can replace the lamb with aubergines/eggplant and sweet potato and replace the lamb stock with vegetable stock. Serve with brown rice or quinoa.

Preparation time: 15 minutes
Cooking time: 2 hours 7 minutes

1 tbsp olive oil or coconut oil
1 onion, sliced
500g/1lb 2oz diced lamb leg steaks
4 tsp harissa paste
400ml/14fl oz/1⅔ cups lamb stock
1 x 400g/14oz can chopped tomatoes
200g/7oz butternut squash chunks (fresh or frozen)
1 carrot, peeled and diced
100g/3½ oz/⅔ cup dried apricots, halved
50g/2oz/½ cup pitted green olives, halved
2 preserved lemons, flesh removed and skin sliced
1 x 400g/14oz can chickpeas/garbanzo beans, drained and rinsed
200g/7oz spinach leaves
handful of coriander/cilantro leaves, chopped
brown rice or quinoa, to serve

1. Preheat the oven to 180°C/350°F/gas mark 4. Heat the oil in a large ovenproof casserole dish and fry the onion and lamb for 5 minutes until browned. Stir in the harissa and cook for 1–2 minutes.
2. Add the stock, tomatoes, vegetables, apricots, olives and lemons and bring to the boil.
3. Transfer the dish to the oven, cover and cook for 1½ hours. Stir in the chickpeas/garbanzo beans, re-cover the dish and cook for a further 30 minutes.
4. Remove from the oven and stir in the spinach leaves – they will wilt in the hot sauce. Serve topped with coriander/cilantro leaves and with either brown rice or quinoa.

Pesto Meatball Pasta Bake

Egg Free
(Nut Free)
Soy Free

These meatballs sneak in vegetables for plenty of flavour, fibre and antioxidants. Frozen peas are a great standby veggie and normally popular with children. They are also packed with fibre and protein, which can help balance blood sugar levels and keep energy levels high. Because they are a good source of fibre they also help keep gut bacteria healthy. You can vary these meatballs by using minced/ground turkey instead of minced/ground lamb, or you could use gluten-free sausages – simply remove the meat from their casings and crumble. The meatballs are also tasty on their own, cold, as an option for lunch boxes.

Preparation time: 20 minutes
Cooking time: 30 minutes

400g/14oz minced/ground lamb
1 small courgette/zucchini, grated
1 shallot, peeled and grated
1 quantity of vegan pesto (see page 196)
olive oil, for drizzling
250g/9oz gluten-free pasta (e.g. penne or fusilli)
2 roasted red peppers (from a jar, drained)
200g/7oz frozen peas
sea salt and freshly ground black pepper

Topping
200g/7oz vegan cheese, grated (check labels), or 200g/7oz/4 cups gluten-free breadcrumbs mixed with 2 tbsp nutritional yeast flakes and 1 tbsp olive oil

1 Preheat the oven to 200°C/400°F/gas mark 6 and lightly grease a baking pan.

2 Place the minced/ground lamb, courgette/zucchini and shallot in a bowl with 1 tbsp pesto and mix together with your hands. Shape into walnut-sized balls and place in the baking pan.

3 Drizzle a little olive oil over the meatballs and bake in the oven for 15 minutes until they are lightly golden.

4 Meanwhile cook the pasta in boiling salted water for 7 minutes or until al dente, stirring occasionally. Drain, reserving 100ml/3½fl oz/scant ½ cup of the cooking water. Return the drained pasta to the saucepan. Stir in the remaining pesto and reserved cooking water. Tip the pasta into an ovenproof dish and stir in the meatballs, red peppers and peas. Season to taste.

5 Sprinkle over the cheese or breadcrumb mixture and return to the oven for 10–15 minutes until the cheese has melted or the crumble topping is lightly golden.

Pulled Jerk Pork

Serves 6

Egg Free
Nut Free
Soy Free

Rubbed with paprika and jerk seasoning then slow-cooked until mouthwateringly tender, this pulled pork is perfect for weekends. Pork is a great source of zinc, a mineral that is essential for the production of stomach acid and the digestive enzymes needed to break down and digest food properly. Good digestion is important to reduce allergic potential and to improve overall gut health. Any leftovers can be added to sandwiches and salads.

Preparation time: 15 minutes
Cooking time: 5 hours 30 minutes

2.5kg/5lb 8oz bone-in pork shoulder joint
2 tbsp jerk seasoning
1 tsp smoked paprika
2 tbsp xylitol
2 tsp sea salt
75ml pineapple juice

To serve

corn tortillas (see page 184) or gluten-free tortillas
fruity salsa (see page 222)
creamy guacamole (see page 283)
shredded lettuce

1. Preheat the oven to 220°C/425°F/gas mark 7.
2. Carefully trim the rind off the shoulder of pork, but leave the fat on. Mix together the jerk seasoning, paprika, xylitol and salt and rub half of it all over the pork shoulder.
3. Place the pork on a rack inside a roasting pan and roast for 30 minutes until it begins to brown.

4 Remove from the oven and reduce the temperature to 150°C/300°F/gas mark 2.
5 Mix the remaining seasoning with the pineapple juice and drizzle over the pork.
6 Pour 200ml/7fl oz/scant 1 cup water into the base of the pan. Cover the pork with a large sheet of foil, sealing it in tightly to prevent steam from escaping.
7 Return to the oven and cook for 5 hours until the meat is meltingly tender.
8 Remove the pork from the oven, keeping it covered with foil. Leave to rest for 20 minutes. Pour the juices from the tray into a bowl.
9 Shred the pork using two forks, discarding any fat, and drizzle with 1–2 tbsp of the reserved cooking juices to keep the meat moist.
10 Warm the tortillas in a cool oven for 1-2 minutes. Spoon some pork, salsa, guacamole and shredded lettuce onto each tortilla and serve as wraps.

Barbecue Traybake Chicken

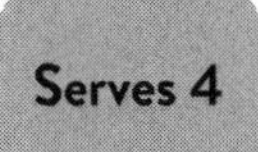

Egg Free

Nut Free

This traybake makes an easy family meal with plenty of colourful vegetables. Onions are a good source of polyphenols that will support the growth of beneficial gut bacteria and of quercetin known for its antihistamine properties. The fruity homemade BBQ sauce is a good accompaniment to a variety of cooked meats and fish. For a vegetarian traybake option you can use a couple of cans of drained and rinsed chickpeas/garbanzo beans instead of the chicken. This recipe uses bone-in chicken thighs but you can use boneless thighs if wished, omitting step 5 and cooking the meat with the vegetables for 30 minutes instead.

Preparation time: 20 minutes
Cooking time: 45 minutes

4 chicken thighs, bone in and skin on
1 tsp fennel seeds
½ tsp smoked paprika
sea salt and freshly ground black pepper
1 tsp xylitol or ½ tsp stevia (optional)
olive oil, for drizzling
1 yellow pepper, deseeded and cut into large chunks
1 red pepper, deseeded and cut into large chunks
1 courgette/zucchini, cut into thick slices
1 red onion, cut into wedges

Barbecue Sauce

1 red onion, diced
1 garlic clove, crushed
1 apple, cored and chopped
60g/2½oz tomato purée/paste
200g/7oz chopped tomatoes
2 tbsp apple cider vinegar
¼ tsp Dijon mustard
1 tbsp xylitol or 1 tsp stevia

1 tbsp tamari (gluten-free soy sauce) (optional)
½ tsp allspice
1 tsp smoked paprika

1. First make the barbecue sauce. Place all the ingredients in a pan and simmer for 15 minutes until the apple is soft and the mixture has thickened. Transfer to a blender and blitz until smooth.
2. Meanwhile preheat the oven to 180°C/350°F/gas mark 4.
3. Place the chicken thighs in a large roasting pan. Blitz the fennel seeds, paprika, salt and pepper and xylitol in a blender or bash using a pestle and mortar until fine.
4. Rub the seasoning all over the chicken then drizzle with a little olive oil.
5. Bake in the oven for 15 minutes.
6. Remove the pan from the oven and scatter over the vegetables. Pour over the sauce and stir to combine.
7. Return the pan to the oven and bake for a further 30 minutes until the chicken is cooked through.

Chicken Schnitzel with Coleslaw

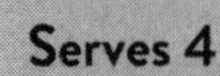

(Egg Free)
(Nut Free)
(Soy Free)

Thin crispy chicken served with a gut-healthy coleslaw makes an easy family evening meal. Fermented foods such as sauerkraut and yogurt provide probiotics, which help modulate our immune response and support a healthy digestive tract. If you don't have any sauerkraut prepared, use 300g/10½oz/4 cups shredded cabbage, and 1 grated carrot and 1 grated apple instead.

Preparation time: 15 minutes
Cooking time: 10-20 minutes

4 small chicken breasts or turkey steaks
4 tbsp cornflour/cornstarch
1 egg, beaten (or use dairy-free yogurt thinned with a little dairy-free milk)
150g/5oz/1½ cups gluten-free breadcrumbs
2 tbsp olive oil
Mixed salad leaves/greens, to serve

Fruity Coleslaw

400g/14oz apple sauerkraut (see page 197), excess liquid drained off
100g/3½oz dairy-free yogurt (see page 194) or mayonnaise (see page 195), or a combination
½ tsp English mustard (optional)

1 Place a chicken breast or turkey steak on a large piece of cling film/plastic wrap, sprinkle with a little water then cover with another piece of cling film/plastic wrap. Beat with a wooden rolling pin until it is nice and thin (about 2–3mm thick. Repeat with the remaining breasts/steaks.

2. Put the cornflour/cornstarch, egg and breadcrumbs on 3 separate plates. Coat each chicken breast first in the cornflour/cornstarch then in egg and finally the breadcrumbs.
3. Heat the oil in a large frying pan and fry the coated chicken for about 5 minutes on each side until brown and cooked through. You may have to do this in batches.
4. Meanwhile make up the coleslaw by mixing all the ingredients together. Serve the chicken with the coleslaw and accompany with a mixed salad.

Moroccan One-pot Chicken with Rice

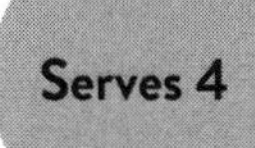

Egg Free
Nut Free
Soy Free

I love one-pot dishes because they mean minimum washing-up and little time spent in the kitchen. You can also prepare this dish ahead of time then simply leave it to cook in the oven when needed. Any leftovers are delicious served cold for lunch the following day. Kale is a 'super green': the carotenoids and magnesium it contains can help reduce allergy symptoms.

Preparation time: 15 minutes
Cooking time: 50 minutes

2 tsp each ground cumin, ground coriander, smoked paprika, ground cinnamon and onion powder
sea salt and freshly ground black pepper
1.5litres/52fl oz/6½ cups chicken stock or homemade bone broth (see page 190)
1 tbsp xylitol or 1 tsp stevia (optional)
1 tbsp olive oil or coconut oil
400g/14oz boneless chicken breast, cut into chunks
1 onion, diced
1 garlic clove, crushed
2 carrots, cut into chunks
300g/10½oz/1½ cups easy-cook brown rice
4 tomatoes, roughly chopped
1 x 400g/14oz can chickpeas/garbanzo beans, drained and rinsed
200g/7oz kale or baby spinach leaves, finely chopped

1. Mix together the spices, salt and pepper, chicken stock and xylitol.
2. Heat the oil in a large ovenproof casserole dish and fry the chicken pieces for 5 minutes until lightly golden. Remove from the pan. Add the onion, garlic and carrots and cook for a further 5 minutes until the onion softens.
3. Tip in the rice and coat in the oil then add the tomatoes and chickpeas/garbanzo beans. Add the chicken back to the pan and pour over the stock. Cover the dish and place in the oven for 40 minutes until the rice is cooked.
4. Remove from the oven and stir in the chopped kale or spinach and allow to wilt for a few minutes before serving.

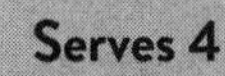

Serves 4

Courgette/Zucchini Noodle Carbonara

This is a lovely healthy twist on the traditional spaghetti carbonara recipe but without any eggs. Using courgette/zucchini noodles is another great way to get your children eating more vegetables, too. The sauce is both egg and dairy free. Garlic and onions are both useful foods for reducing allergy symptoms, including seasonal allergies, as they can help block the production of the chemicals that cause allergic reactions.

Egg Free

Nut Free

Preparation time: 20 minutes
Cooking time: 25 minutes

2 large courgettes/zucchini
2 tsp olive oil
1 shallot, diced
1 garlic clove, crushed
8 streaky bacon slices, diced
sea salt and freshly ground black pepper, to tasste

Sauce

250g/9oz butternut squash
200g/7oz silken tofu, drained
1 tbsp nutritional yeast flakes
1 tbsp tamari (gluten-free soy sauce)
½ tsp cayenne pepper or paprika
juice of ½ lemon
sea salt and freshly ground black pepper, to taste

1 First prepare the courgette/zucchini using a spiralizer to create long noodles. Place in a bowl and set aside.

2 To make the sauce, steam the butternut squash for 10 minutes or until tender. Place all the ingredients in a blender including the squash and blend to form a thick, smooth sauce.
3 Heat the oil in a large sauté pan and fry the shallot, garlic and bacon for about 5 minutes until the bacon is nice and crispy. Toss in the courgette/zucchini noodles and stir for 5 minutes until softened. Pour over the sauce and simmer for 5 minutes to reduce the sauce slightly. Season to taste.
4 Spoon into bowls to serve.

Chowder Fish Pie

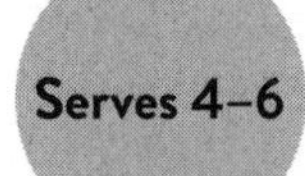

Egg Free
(Nut Free)
(Soy Free)

A mixture of salmon, cod, haddock and prawns/shrimp in a dairy-free creamy sauce and topped with a vegetable mash makes a delicious and nourishing family meal. Omega-3-rich foods such as salmon are one of the most effective foods for lowering inflammation and reducing allergic symptoms, as well as supporting overall brain health and development. This comforting dish can be prepared in advance ready for cooking when needed.

Preparation time: 20 minutes
Cooking time: 38 minutes

600ml/20fl oz/2½ cups dairy-free milk
250g/9oz salmon fillets, skinless, cut into 2.5cm/1in cubes
250g/9oz cod fillets, skinless, cut into 2.5cm/1in cubes
250g/9oz undyed smoked haddock fillets, skinless, cut into 2.5cm/1in cubes
3 tbsp cornflour/cornstarch
150g/5oz cooked prawns/shrimp
200g/7oz can sweetcorn/corn kernels, drained
100g/3½oz frozen peas
2 tbsp freshly chopped chives
sea salt and freshly ground black pepper

Topping
350g/12oz carrots, peeled and cut into chunks
350g/12oz sweet potato, peeled and cut into chunks
1 tbsp dairy-free spread or coconut oil

1. First make the topping by boiling the carrots and sweet potato in a large pan of boiling water for 15 minutes or until tender. Drain, return to the pan and mash with the dairy-free spread.
2. Meanwhile bring the dairy-free milk to the boil in a saucepan, then add the fish cubes (but not the prawns/shrimp). Simmer gently for 2–3 minutes until the fish is cooked through. Transfer the fish to a large bowl using a slotted spoon.
3. Strain the poaching milk into a large jug. Mix the cornflour/cornstarch with 2 tbsp of the poaching milk to form a smooth paste. Add back to the pan and gradually stir in the remaining poaching milk. Return the pan to a medium heat. Bring to a simmer, stirring constantly, and cook for about 5 minutes until thickened.
4. Pour the sauce over the fish and carefully stir in the prawns/shrimp, sweetcorn/corn kernels, peas and chives. Season with salt and pepper. Transfer the mixture to a shallow ovenproof dish (approx. 18cm/7in). Leave to cool then top with the mashed vegetables. You can chill this in the refrigerator if wished and cook when needed.
5. Preheat the oven to 200°C/400°F/gas mark 6.
6. Place the fish pie in the oven and bake for 30 minutes until bubbling round the edges and golden on top.

Fish Bites with Homemade Tomato Ketchup

Serves 4/ makes 8 bites

Nut Free

Soy Free

Make tasty gluten-free fish fingers served with homemade low-sugar ketchup. White fish, such as pollock or cod, is a great source of energy-boosting B vitamins and protein. The crispy oven-baked bites can also be enjoyed cold, so you can pack them into lunch boxes.

Preparation time: 15 minutes
Cooking time: 35 minutes

Fish

250g/9oz pollock, cod or haddock fillets (skinless and boneless)
juice of ½ lemon
50g/2oz/⅓ cup polenta/cornmeal
50g/2oz/½ cup dried gluten-free breadcrumbs (or use an extra 50g/2oz/⅓ cup polenta/cornmeal instead)
sea salt and freshly ground black pepper
1 egg, lightly beaten
2 tbsp olive oil
mixed salad leaves/greens, to serve

Tomato Ketchup

400g/14oz passata
2 tbsp apple cider vinegar
pinch of cayenne pepper
½ tsp garlic powder
½ tsp onion powder
½ tsp ground allspice
2 tbsp xylitol or erythritol
sea salt and freshly ground black pepper

1 First make the ketchup. Put all the ingredients in a pan and bring to the boil, stirring well. Reduce the heat and simmer, uncovered, for about 20 minutes to reduce the sauce until it is quite thick. Stir occasionally to prevent the mixture sticking to the bottom.

2 Leave to cool then store in the refrigerator until required.

3 Preheat the oven to 200°C/400°F/gas mark 6 and grease and line a baking sheet with baking parchment.

4 Cut the fish into 8 pieces, then squeeze over the lemon juice.

5 Mix the polenta/cornmeal and breadcrumbs and season with salt and pepper.

6 Dip the fish into the egg, then turn several times in the polenta/cornmeal mixture to coat. Repeat with all the pieces of fish and lay them on the baking sheet.

7 Drizzle with the olive oil and bake for 15 minutes, turning halfway through cooking.

8 Serve with the ketchup and some steamed vegetables and salad leaves/greens.

Creamy Prawn Tikka Masala

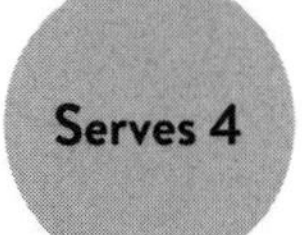

Egg Free
Nut Free
Soy Free

This is a mild and creamy curry with just a little spice. Warm spices can be of real benefit to children with allergies. Ginger is good for the digestion while turmeric is well known for its anti-inflammatory properties, because it contains curcumin, which can block the release of histamine to prevent allergy symptoms from developing. This recipe can be easily adapted if your children are not keen on prawns/shrimp; you could make it with chunks of chicken breast or, for a vegetarian option, replace the seafood with a couple of cans of cooked beans or chickpeas/garbanzo beans.

Preparation time: 20 minutes
Marinating time: 1 hour
Cooking time: 25 minutes

Marinade

2 garlic cloves
2cm/¾in piece root ginger, peeled and roughly chopped
3 tbsp dairy-free yogurt (see page 194)
1 tsp smoked paprika
1 tsp garam masala
½ tsp ground turmeric
2 tsp lemon juice
½ tsp sea salt
450g/1lb raw prawns/shrimp (defrosted if frozen)

Sauce

2 tsp olive oil
1 onion, finely diced
2 garlic cloves, crushed
1 tsp grated root ginger
½ mild red chilli, deseeded and diced
1 tbsp garam masala
¼ tsp ground turmeric
1 carrot, diced

½ red pepper, deseeded and diced
1 x 400g/14oz can peeled plum tomatoes
100ml/3½fl oz/scant ½ cup coconut cream or other dairy-free cream
2 tsp xylitol
100g/3½oz frozen peas
100g/3½oz frozen sliced green beans
handful of fresh coriander/cilantro leaves, chopped

To serve

wholegrain rice or gluten-free naan bread (optional)
mixed salad leaves/greens

1 To make the marinade, purée the garlic and ginger then mix in the yogurt, the paprika, garam masala, turmeric, lemon juice and salt in a glass bowl. Add the prawns/shrimp and stir until coated. Leave to marinate in the refrigerator for 1 hour.

2 To make the sauce, heat the oil in a large saucepan over a low heat. Add the onion and cook gently for about 5 minutes until soft and starting to brown. Add the garlic, ginger and chilli and cook, stirring, for 2 minutes. Stir in the spices, carrot, red pepper, tomatoes, coconut cream and xylitol and break up the tomatoes with a wooden spoon. Simmer for 10–15 minutes until the sauce has thickened. Purée the sauce with a hand-held/immersion blender. Add the peas and green beans and heat through for a couple of minutes.

3 Meanwhile preheat the grill/broiler to high. Remove the prawns from the marinade and place on a lightly greased baking sheet. Grill for 5 minutes, turning halfway through cooking until the prawns/shrimp are pink and slightly golden. Transfer to the curry sauce and mix in.

4 Scatter with chopped coriander/cilantro and serve with rice or gluten-free naan and salad.

Sweet Potato Salmon Fish Cakes

Serves 4

Egg Free
Nut Free
Soy Free

Fish cakes are a great way to sneak in more omega-3-rich fish into your child's diet. You can use canned salmon (without the bones) if you wish but I love the flavour of hot-smoked salmon. Sweet potatoes provide fibre to keep the gut healthy, and are a good source of betacarotene, which the body converts to vitamin A, an important vitamin for immune and gut health. Do include plenty of parsley in the fishcakes; it is rich in anti-allergy nutrients such as carotenoids and vitamin C, and contains apigenin, a flavonoid that has been shown to help lower inflammation and reduce allergy symptoms.

Preparation time: 15 minutes
Cooking time: 20 minutes

400g/14oz sweet potato, peeled and cut into chunks
50g/2oz/½ cup frozen peas
400g/14oz hot-smoked salmon, skin removed
1–2 tsp Thai curry paste or sweet chilli dipping sauce (check labels)
handful of parsley leaves, chopped
50g/2oz/1 cup gluten-free breadcrumbs or gluten-free rolled oats, quinoa flakes or rice cakes
2 tbsp olive oil, for frying

1 Cook the sweet potato in boiling water for 10 minutes or until tender. A couple of minutes before the end of the cooking time add the peas. Drain and mash, allow the mixture to cool slightly.

2 Flake the salmon into the mashed sweet potato and add the curry paste, parsley and breadcrumbs. (If using rice cakes as an alternative to breadcrumbs, process the rice cakes in a food processor roughly first.) Mix well then form the mixture into 4 patties.

3 Heat the olive oil in a frying pan and add the patties. Fry for about 4–5 minutes on each side until crisp and golden.

Oven-baked Mediterranean Risotto

Serves 4

Vegetarian
Vegan
Egg Free
Nut Free
Soy Free

This is a simple vegan dish to prepare and, because it is baked in the oven, the effort involved is minimal. It is full of Mediterranean flavours and red peppers are one of the best vegetable sources of vitamin C, which can help lower histamine and reduce allergy symptoms. For protein, I add a can of beans at the end of cooking.

Preparation time: 15 minutes
Cooking time: 30 minutes

1 tbsp olive oil
1 red onion, chopped
2 garlic cloves, finely chopped
1 courgette/zucchini, diced
300g/10½oz/1½ cups risotto rice
600ml/20fl oz/2½ cups vegetable stock
1 x 400g/14oz can chopped tomatoes
3 roasted red peppers from a jar, drained
1 x 400g/14oz can cannellini or butter/lima beans, drained
handful of parsley leaves, chopped

1 Heat oven to 200°C/400°F/gas mark 6.
2 Heat the oil in large ovenproof casserole dish and fry the onion and garlic for 2–3 minutes until softened. Add the courgette/zucchini and fry for 1 minute, coating the pieces in the oil.
3 Stir in the rice, and fry for a further minute. Pour in the stock, tomatoes and peppers and bring to a simmer, stirring well. Cover the dish and bake in the oven for 25 minutes until the rice is tender and creamy. Stir in the beans and leave to sit for a couple of minutes. Serve topped with the chopped parsley.

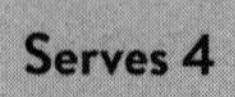

Chunky Veg Stew with Herby Dumplings

Vegetarian
Vegan
Egg Free
(Nut Free)
(Soy Free)

Veg and bean stews make a fabulous family dish on a budget. Carrots, spinach and sweet potato are all great sources of carotenoids and vitamin C to support a healthy immune system.

Preparation time: 20 minutes
Cooking time: 45 minutes

1 tbsp olive oil
1 onion, finely chopped
2 celery stalks, thinly sliced
2 garlic cloves, crushed
1 leek, shredded
1 red chilli, deseeded and diced
300g/10½oz sweet potato, peeled and cut into chunks
2 carrots, peeled and cut into chunks
1 courgette/zucchini, cut into thick slices
1 tsp ground cumin
1 tsp dried thyme
1 x 400g/14oz can chopped tomatoes
600ml/20fl oz/2½ cups vegetable stock
1 x 400g/14oz can butter/lima beans
200g/7oz baby spinach leaves or chopped kale leaves
Sea salt and freshly ground black pepper, to taste

Dumplings

100g/3½oz/1 cup gluten-free flour
1 tsp gluten-free baking powder
50g/2oz chilled dairy-free spread or coconut oil
2 tbsp chopped fresh basil
2 tbsp chopped fresh parsley sea salt and freshly ground black pepper, to taste

1. First make the dumplings. Sift the flour and baking powder into a bowl. Rub in the dairy-free spread to form coarse crumbs and stir in the herbs. Season with salt and pepper. Gradually pour in about 3 tbsp water and combine to form a soft dough. Divide the dough into 12 pieces and roll into balls. Set aside.
2. Heat the oil in a large casserole dish and add the onion, celery, garlic, leek and red chilli. Cook over a low heat for 10 minutes until the leek and celery have softened. Add the sweet potato, carrots, courgette/zucchini, cumin and thyme and cook for a further 5 minutes.
3. Stir in the tomatoes, stock and beans and bring to the boil. Reduce the heat and drop in the dumplings. Cover the dish and simmer for 30 minutes or until the dumplings are puffed up. Add the spinach or kale and gently stir for a couple of minutes until wilted. Season to taste.
4. Serve in bowls. It is delicious topped with a little dairy-free yogurt (see page 194).

Smoky Bean Burgers

Makes 4 large or 8 small burgers

Vegetarian
Vegan
Egg Free
Nut Free
Soy Free

These vegan burgers are packed with flavour and are delicious served with barbecue sauce or homemade tomato ketchup. Serve in gluten-free rolls or simply accompany with salad leaves/greens and fruity coleslaw. Kidney beans provide plenty of protein and oats are a source of soluble fibre to help stabilize blood sugar levels. You can also use gluten-free breadcrumbs instead of rolled oats or swap for quinoa, millet or buckwheat flakes.

Preparation time: 20 minutes
Cooking time: 10 minutes

1 x 400g/14oz can red kidney beans, rinsed and drained
75g/3oz/¾ cup gluten-free rolled oats or gluten-free dried breadcrumbs or quinoa flakes
sea salt and freshly ground black pepper, to taste, to taste

Spice Paste

2 garlic cloves, chopped
1 small onion, chopped
1 tomato, chopped
2 tbsp tomato purée/paste or homemade tomato ketchup (see page 255)
1 tbsp olive oil
2 tsp xylitol
2 tsp ground cumin
1 tsp smoked paprika
pinch of chilli powder
2 tbsp ground flaxseed

To serve

mixed salad leaves/greens
fruity coleslaw (see page 247)
homemade tomato ketchup (see page 255) or barbecue sauce (see page 245)

1. Put all the ingredients for the spice paste in a food processor and process to form a thick paste. Add the beans and gluten-free oats and blend briefly to combine everything but keep some texture. Season with salt and pepper.
2. Divide the mixture into 4 large or 8 small burgers, then wet your hands and shape into burgers. The burgers can now be frozen if wished.
3. To cook preheat the grill/broiler to high. Place on a non-stick baking sheet, then grill/broil for 5 minutes on each side until golden and crisp. To cook the burgers from frozen, bake in the oven at 200°C/400°F/gas mark 6 for 20–30 minutes until cooked through and lightly brown.
4. Serve with salad, coleslaw and ketchup or barbecue sauce.

Harissa Traybake Vegetables and Chickpeas with Herby Yogurt

Serves 4

Vegetarian
Vegan
Egg Free
(Nut Free)
(Soy Free)

Roasting vegetables gives them a wonderful sweetness that children love. You can serve this from the oven or cold as a salad. Either way, the dish is full of antioxidant-rich vegetables and the dressing made with yogurt introduces probiotics to support a healthy gut and immune system.

Preparation time: 15 minutes
Cooking time: 40 minutes

1 medium sweet potato (350g/12oz) peeled and cut into 1cm chunks
2 red onions, cut into large chunks
1 red pepper, deseeded and cut into large pieces
1 yellow pepper, deseeded and cut into large pieces
2 courgettes/zucchini, cut into large slices
4 tbsp olive oil
2 tsp balsamic vinegar
sea salt and freshly ground black pepper, to taste
2 tsp harissa paste
juice of ½ lemon
1 tsp xylitol
1 x 400g/14oz can chickpeas/garbanzo beans, drained

Yogurt Dressing

200ml/7fl oz/scant 1 cup dairy-free yogurt (see page 194)
1 tbsp lemon juice
sea salt and freshly ground black pepper, to taste
15g chopped fresh mint

1 Preheat the oven to 200°C/400°F/gas mark 6. Arrange the vegetables in a large roasting pan and drizzle with 2 tbsp oil and the vinegar and season with salt and pepper. Roast in the oven for 30 minutes, turning the vegetables once to ensure they roast evenly.

2 Mix the harissa paste with the lemon juice, xylitol and remaining oil. Remove the roasting pan from the oven, stir in the chickpeas/garbanzo beans and harissa dressing and return to the oven for a further 10 minutes.

3 To make the yogurt dressing simply mix the ingredients together in a bowl and chill until required.

4 Spoon the vegetables onto plates and top with yogurt dressing to serve.

Desserts

Just because your child has allergies does not mean they have to miss out on dessert. Unlike traditional puddings and desserts these options are low in added sugars yet packed with flavour and nutrients. These sweet treats include a combination of vegetables, fruits and plenty of healthy fats and protein. With a great range of options these will be enjoyed by the whole family and you would never know they are allergy free.

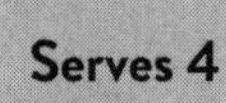

Speedy Banana Ice Cream with Chocolate Sauce

Ice cream made with frozen bananas is a fabulous way to give your children a healthy and allergy-free treat. Slice peeled ripe bananas and freeze on a tray until firm and keep in sealed bags in the freezer ready to make your ice cream. There are many ways to flavour the basic recipe, and I have given various suggestions below. Try serving it drizzled with chocolate sauce (see opposite).

Vegetarian
Vegan
Egg Free
(Nut Free)
(Soy Free)

Preparation time 10 minutes
Freezing time (optional) 30 minutes

Basic Recipe

3 bananas peeled, sliced and frozen
1–2 tbsp dairy-free milk (as needed)

1. Put the frozen banana slices in a food processor or high speed blender and blend until you achieve a consistency that resembles soft serve. If your blender is having trouble processing, add 1–2 tbsp dairy-free milk.
2. Once the soft-serve texture is reached, you can serve it immediately or, for a firmer texture, scoop the ice cream into a container and freeze for 30 minutes or so, then scoop out with an ice cream scoop.

Chocolate Banana Ice Cream: Add ½ tsp pure vanilla extract and 2–3 tbsp unsweetened cocoa powder.

Mint Chocolate Chip: Add a few drops of pure peppermint extract and stir in dairy-free chocolate chips after blending. If you want it to look green, add a pinch of spirulina powder when blending.

Berry: Add 150g frozen berries of your choice and ½ tsp pure vanilla extract.

Piña Colada: Use 3 tbsp coconut cream (in place of the dairy-free milk) and blend in 100g/3½oz frozen pineapple chunks.

Chocolate Sauce

100ml/3½fl oz/scant ½ cup water

50g/2oz/½ cup unsweetened cocoa powder or cacao powder

1–3 tsp maple syrup or other sweetener, to taste

30g/1oz cacao butter or dairy-free chocolate, broken into pieces

1 tsp pure vanilla extract

1 Mix a little of the water into the cacao powder to make a thin paste. Then put all the ingredients in a small pan over a low heat and bring to a gentle simmer, whisking all the time.

2 Allow the mixture to simmer gently while whisking for 5 minutes until it has thickened slightly. Serve immediately or chill and store in the refrigerator. You can reheat the sauce with a little extra dairy-free milk when needed.

Green Ice Lollies/Popsicles

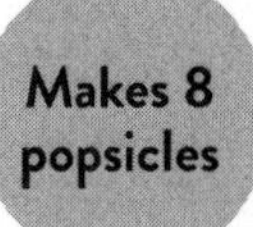

Vegetarian
Vegan
Egg Free
Soy Free

Blending nutrient-rich spinach with sweet mango and banana is a fun way to encourage your children to enjoy greens. Bananas are a great source of gut-healthy fibre to support beneficial bacteria. Mango provides vitamin C and carotenoids, which are particularly beneficial for a healthy respiratory tract. These lollies/popsicles contain avocado to provide plenty of anti-inflammatory monounsaturated fats.

Preparation time 15 minutes
Freezing time: 2 hours

1 ripe banana
50g/2oz/1 cup spinach leaves
½ avocado, pitted
175g/6oz/1 cup frozen mango
125ml/4fl oz/½ cup coconut water
125ml/4fl oz/½ cup coconut milk

Blend all the ingredients in a blender until smooth. Pour the mixture into 8 lolly/popsicle moulds/molds and freeze for about 2 hours until firm.

Tropical Parfait

Serves 4

Vegetarian
Vegan
Egg Free
(Nut Free)
Soy Free

This is such a quick and simple dessert and ideal as a breakfast option, too. Layers of gluten-free granola, probiotic-rich yogurt and tropical fruit are sure to go down well. Any fruit, including frozen fruit, works, making this an easy standby recipe to put together.

Preparation time: 15 minutes

300g/10½oz mango flesh, cut into small pieces (about 1 large fruit)
300g/10½oz pineapple, cut into small pieces
15g chia seeds
200g/7oz/2 cups homemade granola (see page 200) or gluten-free rolled oats, toasted (or you can use millet flakes, rice flakes or buckwheat flakes)
200g/7oz dairy-free yogurt (see page 194) or thick coconut cream (simply remove the thick cream from the top of a chilled can of full-fat coconut milk)

1 Mix the fruit together in a bowl. Transfer half of the mix to a blender, add the chia seeds and blend to a purée. Leave the mixture to stand for 5 minutes then blitz again – it will have thickened slightly.
2 Spoon a little granola or oats in the base of four glasses. Top with a little fruit purée then a little yogurt or coconut cream and finally a little chopped fruit. Repeat the layers, finishing with the chopped fruit.

Easy Chocolate Mousse

This chocolate mousse is naturally sweetened with orange rather than sugars or syrups. Cacao powder is rich in antioxidants and has been found to have anti-allergy properties because it helps to reduce the synthesis of immunoglobulin E (IgE) associated with allergies. It can support the growth of healthy gut bacteria, too. Depending on your child's allergies, you can either use dairy-free yogurt or silken tofu for the creamy texture.

Vegetarian
Vegan
Egg Free
Nut Free
Soy Free

Preparation time: 10 minutes
Cooking time: 3 minutes
Chilling time: 1 hour

150g dairy-free chocolate, broken into pieces
1 tbsp dairy-free milk
2 tbsp unsweetened cocoa powder or cacao powder
2 small oranges, peeled
250g thick dairy-free yogurt (see page 194) or silken tofu
orange segments to decorate (or mandarin segments from a can)

1 Put the chocolate and milk in a pan over a low heat and gently melt, stirring to combine.
2 Put the melted chocolate into a blender with all the remaining ingredients, except the orange segments and blend until smooth and creamy.
3 Pour into individual ramekins or glasses and chill for 1 hour to set. Decorate with the orange segments before serving.

Strawberry Jam Mug Cake

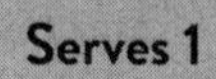

Vegetarian
Vegan
(Egg Free)
(Nut Free)
(Soy Free)

This is a fun treat made in the microwave for a speedy option, although you can cook it in the oven, too. Choose a pure fruit spread with no added sugars for the jam. Top with some dairy-free yogurt for a probiotic boost. You can make it egg free by using flaxseed.

Preparation time: 5 minutes
Cooking time: 2 minutes

1 tbsp xylitol
1 tbsp olive oil or melted dairy-free spread
1 egg (or flax egg made with 1 tbsp ground flaxseed and 3 tbsp water)
2 tbsp dairy-free milk
½ tsp vanilla extract
4 tbsp gluten-free plain/all-purpose flour
½ tsp gluten-free baking powder
1 tbsp strawberry jam (no added sugar)

dairy-free yogurt, to serve (optional)

1. Put all the ingredients except the jam in a microwave-safe (or ovenproof) mug and mix well with a fork until smooth. Place the strawberry jam in the middle of the mixture, pushing it down into the batter. Microwave on high for 2 minutes. Serve with a spoonful of dairy-free yogurt.
2. To bake in the oven, preheat the oven to 180°C/350°F/gas mark 4.
3. Bake for 15 minutes until cooked and golden.

Berry Apple Crumble

Serves 4

Vegetarian
Vegan
Egg Free
Nut Free
Soy Free

Crumble is the ideal comfort food. Oats are a source of soluble fibre, which is easy to digest and stabilizes blood sugar levels. If your child cannot tolerate oats, use quinoa, rice or buckwheat flakes instead. Serve this with dairy-free yogurt or dairy-free custard.

Preparation time: 15 minutes
Cooking time: 23 minutes

3 apples, cored and chopped
250g frozen mixed berries

Crumble Topping

200g/7oz/2 cups gluten-free rolled oats, quinoa flakes, rice flakes or buckwheat flakes
50g/2oz/½ cup gluten-free plain/all-purpose flour
1 tsp ground cinnamon
1 tbsp maple syrup
2 tbsp apple juice
2 tbsp olive oil or melted coconut oil
1 tsp vanilla extract

1. Preheat the oven to 180°C/350°F/gas mark 4.
2. Make the topping. Place all the ingredients in a bowl and mix thoroughly together.
3. Put the apples and berries in a pan with 1 tbsp water and heat gently. Cover and simmer gently for 2–3 minutes until the apples are beginning to soften.
4. Spoon the fruit into a 18cm/7in baking dish. Sprinkle over the crumble topping. Bake in the oven for 20 minutes until the crumble is lightly golden and the fruit is bubbling.

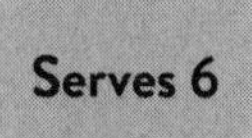

Baked Rice Pudding with Spiced Plum Compôte

Vegetarian
Vegan
Egg Free
(Nut Free)
(Soy Free)

This is a deliciously healthier version of traditional rice pudding. Using wholegrain brown rice provides B vitamins for energy, soluble fibre and slow-releasing carbohydrates. The addition of coconut milk gives it a creamy texture and is a source of lauric acid to boost immune health and caprylic acid, known to support gut health. If you cannot tolerate coconut, though, simply use another dairy-free milk and spread.

Preparation time: 15 minutes
Cooking time: 53 minutes

1 tbsp coconut oil or dairy-free spread
150g/5oz/¾ cup brown rice
1 tbsp xylitol
2 x 400g/14oz cans full-fat coconut milk
1 tsp vanilla extract
1 tsp ground cinnamon
1 tbsp ground flaxseed
200ml/7fl oz/scant 1 cup water

Spiced Plum Compôte

250g plums, pitted and chopped
1 tbsp xylitol
1 tbsp water
2 star anise

1 Preheat the oven to 180°C/350°F/gas mark 4.
2 Heat the coconut oil or dairy-free spread in a large ovenproof dish and add the rice. Stir to coat the grains in the oil for 2–3 minutes to create a nutty flavour.

3 Add the xylitol, coconut milk, vanilla extract, cinnamon, flaxseed and water. Bring to the boil and stir well. Transfer the dish to the oven and bake for 50 minutes until the rice is very tender and most of the liquid has been absorbed.

4 Meanwhile make the compôte. Put the plums and the other ingredients in a small pan over a low heat. Stir well and simmer gently for 5 minutes until the plums are very soft, breaking them up with a wooden spoon. Remove the star anise.

5 Spoon the rice pudding into bowls and top with a little of the plum compôte.

Gooey Lemon Dessert

Serves 4

Vegetarian
(Nut Free)
(Soy Free)

This self-saucing dessert takes little effort to prepare. The result is warming, gooey and tangy. Lemons are a great source of limonene, found in lemon zest, and vitamin C, which can help lessen allergy symptoms.

Preparation time: 15 minutes
Cooking time: 40 minutes

125g/4½oz/1 cup gluten-free plain/all-purpose flour
1 tsp gluten-free baking powder
75g/3oz/¾ cup xylitol
1 egg
50g/2oz melted dairy-free spread or coconut oil
100ml/3½fl oz/scant ½ cup dairy-free milk
zest and juice of 2 lemons
1 tbsp cornflour/cornstarch
1 tbsp custard powder (check labels)

1. Preheat the oven to 180°C/350°F/gas mark 4.
2. Combine the flour, baking powder and half the xylitol in a bowl.
3. Add the egg, melted spread, dairy-free milk and lemon zest and beat to combine.
4. Pour the batter into an 18cm/7in ovenproof dish.
5. Combine the cornflour/cornstarch, custard powder and the remaining xylitol in a jug. Carefully blend in the lemon juice to form a smooth paste. Then add 375ml/13fl oz/1½ cups boiling water. Pour over the batter and immediately place in the oven.
6. Bake for 30–40 minutes or until puffed and golden. Serve warm, with dairy-free yogurt, if wished.

Savoury Snacks

Children of all ages love coming home to a snack – whether it's to bridge the gap between breakfast and lunch, to perk them up during the after-school slump, or to raise energy levels after a sporting activity. A healthy snack can provide your child with key nutrients, as well as stabilizing blood sugar levels to keep them energized. Keeping it simple and natural, rather than resorting to processed supermarket offerings, is the best approach and with a little planning it is easy to make your own tasty options ahead of time. Many of these snacks can also be made by the children themselves, providing a perfect opportunity to develop more independence and control over their diets. I have included both sweet and savoury options to suit all tastes.

Buckwheat Seed Crackers

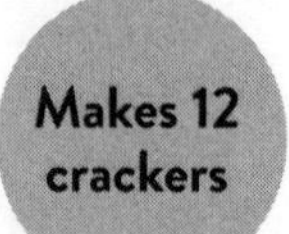

Egg Free
(Nut Free)
(Soy Free)

Many shop-bought crackers are low in fibre and high in salt. This recipe offers a healthy alternative that is perfect as a snack or served with dips. Flaxseed and chia seeds are a useful vegetarian source of omega-3 fats as well as providing plenty of fibre for a healthy gut. You can vary the seeds according to taste.

Preparation time: 20 minutes
Cooking time: 20 minutes

100g/3½oz/1 cup buckwheat flour
50g/2oz/½ cup gluten-free plain/all-purpose flour
½ tsp gluten-free baking powder
1 tbsp ground flaxseed or chia seeds
1 tsp garlic salt
1 tsp chopped fresh rosemary
60ml/2½fl oz olive oil or melted dairy-free spread
about 3 tbsp water, to mix
2 tbsp sesame seeds, sunflower seeds and poppy seeds, plus extra for sprinkling

1 Preheat the oven to 180°C/350°F/gas mark 4 and grease a large baking sheet.
2 Put the flours, baking powder, flaxseed, salt and rosemary in a food processor and process briefly to combine. Add the olive oil or dairy-free spread and mix well. Add in a little water to form a soft dough. Add the seeds and pulse in briefly to mix.
3 Place the dough between two sheets of cling film/plastic wrap and roll out to about 3mm/⅛ in thick. Cut out circles with a small cookie cutter about 6cm/2½in and place the crackers

on the baking sheet. Brush the tops with a little water and sprinkle over a few more seeds.

4 Bake in the oven for 15–20 minutes until golden. Leave to cool for 5 minutes before transferring to a wire/cooling rack.

5 These crackers can be kept in an airtight container for 3–4 days. You can also freeze the crackers and the unbaked dough.

Vegetable Crisps

Vegetarian
Vegan
Egg Free
Nut Free
Soy Free

These colourful crisps are a great way to give your kids root vegetables. Tubers and root vegetables are useful sources of fibre to support healthy digestion and encourage a greater diversity of healthy gut bacteria. Because these crisps are oven-baked, not deep-fried, they are much healthier than many shop-bought versions.

Preparation time: 15 minutes
Cooking time: 15 minutes

1 beetroot/beet
1 sweet potato
1 parsnip
2 tbsp olive oil
½ teaspoon salt or garlic salt
½ teaspoon xylitol or stevia (optional)
¼ tsp smoked paprika
¼ tsp ground cumin

1. Preheat the oven to 200°C/400°F/gas mark 6. Line a couple of baking sheets with baking parchment. Trim the ends from the vegetables, then wash but don't peel them.
2. Mix together the olive oil with the spices.
3. Using a sharp knife or mandolin, slice all the vegetables into very thin rounds. Press between paper towels or a clean dish towel to dry off excess moisture. Put the slices in a bowl and pour over the spiced oil. Stir to coat thoroughly.
4. Spread out the slices in a single layer on the baking sheets and bake in the oven for about 15 minutes or until golden. Remove from the oven and leave to cool. The crisps can be stored in an airtight container for 1–2 days – they will crisp up again if you heat them in a warm oven for a few minutes.

Creamy Guacamole

Serves 4

Vegetarian
Vegan
Egg Free
Nut Free
Soy Free

Guacamole, with its creamy flavour, sharpened with lime and a hint of chilli, is a popular dip for raw vegetable sticks or as a spread for breads and crackers. Avocados are rich in healthy monounsaturated fats and have high levels of vitamin E, iron and potassium as well as antioxidants including lutein, a carotenoid that improves skin conditions. Cool and smooth textured, avocados are a wonderful anti-inflammatory food. This chunky dip combines this superfruit with onion, tomato and probiotic-rich yogurt.

Preparation time: 15 minutes

1 ripe avocado, pitted and diced
2 tbsp dairy-free yogurt (see page 194)
¼ red onion, diced
1 tablespoon chopped fresh coriander/cilantro
1 ripe tomato, diced
½ red chilli, deseeded and diced
2 tsp lime juice
sea salt and freshly ground pepper, to taste

1 Mash the avocado with a fork in a bowl. Add the remaining ingredients and mix well to form a chunky dip.
2 Season with salt and pepper to taste. Best served immediately.

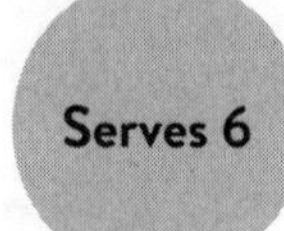

Spicy Chickpeas

Vegetarian
Vegan
Egg Free
Nut Free
Soy Free

This is a fabulously healthy protein-rich snack that makes a useful alternative to nuts. You can vary the flavours according to your own child's tastes.

Preparation time: 5 minutes
Cooking time: 30 minutes

1 x 400g/14oz can chickpeas/ garbanzo beans, drained
1 tsp olive oil
1 tsp smoked paprika
1 tsp ground cumin
1 tsp ground coriander/cilantro

1. Preheat the oven to 180°C/350°F/gas mark 4.
2. Dry the chickpeas/garbanzo beans in a clean dish towel then tip into a bowl. Toss in the oil and spices and mix well until the chickpeas/garbanzo beans are well coated.
3. Tip out onto a baking sheet and bake for about 30 minutes, or until they're crunchy moving them round halfway through so they dry out evenly. Leave to cool, then store in an airtight container.

Sweet Treats

In this section you will find a wonderful selection of healthy sweet treats. Ideal for after school or packed lunches, these are also perfect for parties, too. Unlike traditional cookies and cakes, these recipes focus on keeping the sugar low while cramming in many nourishing ingredients.

Ginger Oaty Cookies

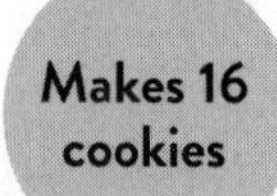

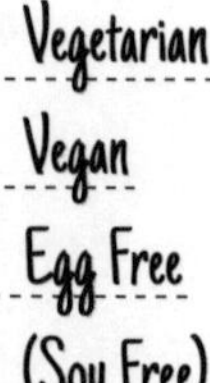

These chunky cookies are a lovely lunch box filler or after school treat. Ginger is a natural antihistamine and can help lower the production of immunoglobulin E (IgE), antibodies associated with seasonal allergies like hay fever.

Preparation time: 15 minutes
Cooking time: 20 minutes

30g/1oz coconut flour
30g/1oz tapioca flour
30g/1oz arrowroot powder
1 tbsp xylitol
30g/1oz gluten-free rolled oats (or use quinoa or rice flakes)
1 tsp gluten-free baking powder
½ tsp ground ginger
½ tsp bicarbonate of soda/baking soda
1 tbsp ground flaxseed
60ml/2½ fl oz melted coconut oil or dairy-free spread
2 pieces of stem ginger, diced
3–4 tbsp syrup from the stem ginger jar

1. Preheat the oven to 180°C/350°F/gas mark 4. Grease and line a baking sheet with baking parchment.
2. Put the flours, arrowroot, xylitol, oats, baking powder, ginger, bicarbonate of soda/baking soda and flaxseed in a food processor and blend together to break up the oats lightly. Add the melted oil, stem ginger and syrup and process to form a soft dough. Roll the dough into walnut-size balls and place, spaced apart, on the baking sheet. Press down on top of each ball with a fork to form small rounds.
3. Bake for 20 minutes or until lightly golden.
4. Transfer to a wire/cooling rack to cool completely.

Lemon Chia Shortbread

Makes 16 shortbreads

Vegetarian
Vegan
Egg Free
(Nut Free)
(Soy Free)

This is a melt-in-the-mouth lemon shortbread that no one has to resist. By using xylitol, you can keep the sugar content low while the addition of chia seeds provides additional fibre, protein and essential omega-3 fats.

Preparation time: 20 minutes
Chilling time: 30 minutes
Cooking time: 45 minutes

250g/9oz/2¼ cups gluten-free plain/all-purpose flour
1 tsp xanthum gum
1 tsp gluten-free baking powder
60g/2½oz/½ cup xylitol
175g/6oz chilled dairy-free spread, cubed
zest of 2 lemons and juice of ½ lemon
30g/1oz chia seeds

1. Grease a baking sheet and line with baking parchment.
2. Put the flour, xanthan gum, baking powder and xylitol in a food processor and process to combine.
3. Add the dairy-free spread and lemon zest. Pulse to mix thoroughly. Add the chia seeds and lemon juice and process again to form a soft dough.
4. Wrap the dough in cling film/plastic wrap and chill for 30 minutes to firm up.
5. Preheat the oven to 180°C/350°F/gas mark 4.
6. Place the dough on a sheet of baking parchment and lightly roll out to form a rectangle about 3mm/⅛in thick.

7 Carefully lift the dough onto the baking sheet. Cut the dough with a knife into 16 equal pieces. Press the prongs of a fork evenly over the dough.

8 Bake for 20 minutes then remove from the oven and cut again through the original lines. This will ensure the shortbread slices remain separate on cooking.

9 Return the shortbread to the oven and bake for a further 25 minutes until golden.

10 Remove the shortbread from the oven and leave to cool on the sheet for 20 minutes before transferring to a wire/cooling rack to cool completely.

11 The shortbread can be stored in an airtight container for 5–7 days.

Orange Polenta Traybake

Makes a 20cm/8in traybake

Vegetarian
(Vegan)
(Egg Free)
(Nut Free)
(Soy Free)

In the spirit of a lemon drizzle cake, but with a healthy orange syrup instead of a sugary crust, this moist dessert cake is baked in a traybake pan and cut into squares. Polenta/cornmeal makes a deliciously dense cake to serve with dairy-free yogurt or ice cream. The syrup is poured over the cake as soon as it comes out the oven for a lovely sticky glaze. To make this egg free substitute the eggs for 150g/5oz apple puree with ½ tsp xanthum gum and increase the baking powder to 2 tsp.

Preparation time: 15 minutes
Cooking time: 40 minutes

Cake

200g/7oz dairy-free spread or coconut oil
100g/3½oz/1 cup xylitol
3 eggs
2 tsp vanilla extract
1 tbsp orange juice
zest of 2 oranges
150g/5oz/1½ cups gluten-free plain/all-purpose flour
150g/5oz/1 cup fine polenta/cornmeal
1 tsp gluten-free baking powder
½ tsp bicarbonate of soda/baking soda

Orange Syrup

juice of 3 oranges
3 tbsp xylitol

1 Preheat the oven to 180°C/350°F/gas mark 4. Grease a square 20cm/8in shallow traybake pan and line with baking parchment.

2 Place the dairy-free spread in a food processor with the xylitol and beat until light and creamy.
3 Gradually beat in the eggs and vanilla extract, orange juice and zest. Slowly add the remaining ingredients and combine to form a smooth batter.
4 Spoon the batter into the traybake pan. Bake for 35 minutes or until the cake is golden and when a skewer is inserted into the middle it comes out clean.
5 Meanwhile make the syrup. Place the juice and xylitol in a small saucepan and simmer gently to dissolve the xylitol, about 3 minutes.
6 Prick the warm cake all over with a skewer and pour over the syrup.
7 Leave to cool then cut into squares to serve.

Chocolate Layered Cream Cake

Serves 8/makes a 15cm/6in cake

Vegetarian
Vegan
Egg Free
(Nut Free)
(Soy Free)

This is a wonderful rich vegan cake that's perfect for birthdays and celebrations. If your child cannot eat coconut you could use soy yogurt (strained) or omit and simply layer with the jam.

Preparation time: 30 minutes
Chilling time: 24 hours
Cooking time: 30 minutes

Cake

250g/9oz/2¼ cups gluten-free plain/all-purpose flour
1 tsp bicarbonate of soda/baking soda
1 tsp gluten-free baking powder
50g/2oz/½ cup unsweetened cocoa powder
100ml/3½fl oz/scant ½ cup olive oil
125g/4½ oz/1¼ cups xylitol or erythritol
180g/6oz apple purée
225ml/8fl oz/scant 1 cup dairy-free milk
1 tsp lemon juice
sugar-free berry jam

Coconut Cream (optional)

60ml/2fl oz aquafaba (the thick liquid from a can of chickpeas/garbanzo beans)
1 tbsp xylitol
¼ tsp xanthan gum
60g/2oz coconut cream (the thick cream from a can of full-fat coconut milk)

Chocolate Ganache

115g dairy-free chocolate, grated or chopped
100ml/3½fl oz/scant ½ cup dairy-free cream or coconut cream

1. First make the coconut cream. Pour the aquafaba into a large glass bowl. Using an electric whisk beat the liquid until it forms soft peaks (similar to whisking up egg whites); this may take up to 10 minutes. Gradually add the xylitol and whisk it in, then add the xanthum gum. Very slowly whisk in the coconut cream until smooth. Place in the refrigerator for at least 4 hours or ideally overnight to thicken.
2. Preheat the oven to 180°C/350°F/gas mark 4. Grease and line with baking parchment three shallow 15cm/6in round baking pans.
3. Put the flour, bicarbonate of soda/baking soda, baking powder and cocoa powder in a food processor and process together.
4. In a separate bowl whisk the remaining ingredients except the jam or blend in a blender.
5. Gradually add the wet ingredients to the food processor and blend to form a smooth batter.
6. Divide the batter between the greased pans. Bake the cakes for about 30 minutes or until risen and firm to touch.
7. Cool in the pans for 10 minutes then turn out onto a wire/cooling rack and remove the baking parchment. Leave to cool completely before frosting.
8. Make the ganache. Put the chocolate and cream in a saucepan over a low heat and heat gently, stirring all the time, until thick. Leave to cool slightly until it has a thick coating consistency.
9. To assemble, spread some of the jam on one of the cake layers then top with a little of the chilled coconut cream. Place a second cake layer on top and repeat with the jam and coconut cream. Top with the remaining cake layer and spread the surface with the chocolate ganache.
10. Store the cake in the refrigerator until required.

Sweet Potato Brownies

Makes 16 brownies

Vegetarian
(Nut Free)
(Soy Free)

Few can resist a rich gooey chocolate brownie and no one would guess this version contains sweet potato! This makes a lovely family treat and it's perfect for children's parties, too. Sweet potatoes are a great source of soluble fibre to support healthy gut bacteria and they provide plenty of carotenoids to help modulate the immune system and support a healthy gut lining.

Preparation time: 15 minutes
Cooking time: 1 hour

1 medium sweet potato (200g/7oz)
100g/3½oz dairy-free spread, cubed
200g/7oz dairy-free chocolate, chopped
80g/3¼oz/¾ cup xylitol
2 eggs, beaten
2 tsp vanilla extract
100g/3½oz/1 cup gluten-free plain/all-purpose flour
1 tsp gluten-free baking powder
30g/1oz unsweetened cocoa powder
75g/3oz/¾ cup dairy-free chocolate chips or dried cherries

1 Preheat the oven to 190°C/375°F/gas mark 5. Grease a square 20cm baking pan and line with baking parchment.

2 Prick the sweet potato then bake in the oven for 35 minutes or until soft. Leave to cool then remove the skin and place the flesh in a food processor.

3 Put the dairy-free spread, chocolate and xylitol in a saucepan over a low heat to melt, stirring regularly.

4. Pour the chocolate mixture into the food processor then add the sweet potato and blend until smooth. Tip in the eggs, vanilla, flour, baking powder and cocoa powder and process to form a stiff batter.
5. Pulse in the chocolate chips or dried cherries.
6. Spoon the mixture into the lined pan and smooth the surface.
7. Bake in the oven for 25 minutes until firm on top.
8. Leave to cool before cutting into bars.

Malt Loaf

Makes 1 loaf/about 10 slices

Vegetarian
Vegan
Egg Free
Nut Free
Soy Free

This is a gluten-free, dairy-free and egg-free version of the popular malt loaf. Perfect as a sweet treat after school. Ideally, wrap the loaf in greaseproof paper and leave for a day before eating as the loaf becomes even more sticky.

Preparation time: 15 minutes
Soaking time: 30 minutes
Cooking time: 45 minutes

200ml/7fl oz/scant 1 cup black tea
4 tbsp maple syrup or yacón syrup
4 tbsp apple purée
2 tbsp black strap molasses
200g/7oz/1½ cups raisins
175g/6oz/scant 2 cups gluten-free plain/all-purpose flour (or see page 182)
60g/2½oz/½ cup buckwheat flour
1 tsp xanthan gum
1 tbsp baking powder
pinch of sea salt

1. Put the tea, syrup, apple purée, molasses and raisins in a bowl and leave to soak for 30 minutes.
2. Preheat the oven to 180°C/350°F/gas mark 4. Grease a 450g/1lb loaf pan and line with baking parchment.
3. Put the flours, xanthan gum, baking powder and salt in a food processor, and process briefly to combine.
4. Pour in the tea mixture and process until it forms a thick, sticky batter.

5. Pour the batter into the prepared tin and bake for about 40–45 minutes, until a skewer inserted into the middle of the loaf comes out clean.
6. Remove from the oven and leave to cool in the tin.
7. Once cold wrap in greaseproof paper and store in an airtight container. The cake will keep for 2–3 days or can be frozen for up to a month.

Resources

Functional Lab Testing and Healthcare Practitioner Support

Various laboratories in the UK, US and other countries offer IgG food tests. They are all blood tests. Some of these can be undertaken at home while others require a blood draw. Many of these are only available through healthcare practitioners or qualified registered nutritional consultants.

YorkTest Laboratories

yorktest.com

YorkTest provide a Home Spot blood test to the UK and most states of the US (at the time of printing, excluding New York, New Jersey, Maryland and Rhode Island), to identify IgG food reactions.

Cyrex Laboratory

cyrexlabs.com

Available only through qualified practitioners, Cyrex™ is a US-based Clinical Immunology Laboratory specializing in autoimmunity and food reactions. Various tests are available which include gluten testing, multiple food testing and cross-reactive food testing. A full blood draw is required.

Vitamin and Mineral Tests, Intestinal Permeability, Breath Tests and Stool Testing

Doctors and qualified practitioners can order a wide range of functional laboratory tests based on the individual's needs.

British Association for Nutrition and Lifestyle Medicine (BANT)

bant.org.uk

BANT is a professional body for Registered Nutrition Practitioners. You can search for a practitioner via the website.

Institute of Functional Medicine (IFM)

ifm.org

The IFM provides education and training in functional medicine. For a registered practitioner trained in functional medicine, visit the website.

Charities, Organizations and Support Sites

IN THE UK

Action Against Allergy

actionagainstallergy.org

National charity providing help, support and advice through forums, articles, newsletters and events.

Allergy Lifestyle

allergylifestyle.com

This online shop ships worldwide, and provides resources and equipment for those with allergy, asthma and anaphylaxis.

Allergy UK

allergyuk.org

Allergy UK is a charity supporting people with allergies and chemical sensitivities. Their website contains a wide range of information and resources.

Anaphylaxis Campaign

anaphylaxis.org.uk

Excellent support group for anyone suffering from a severe food allergy.

Asthma UK

asthma.org.uk

The UK's leading asthma charity, with a very informative website.

Coeliac UK

coeliac.org.uk

This is the UK's national charity for coeliac disease, and helps people living without gluten. They provide a wealth of information and resources to help people manage their health and diet including recipes, parental support, and a gluten-free checker app for help when shopping.

Foods Matter

foodsmatter.com

This independent informational series of websites provides information on coeliac disease and gluten-related disorders, free-from food, free-from supplements, free-from recipes and allergic skin conditions.

National Eczema Society

eczema.org

The UK's national eczema charity, dedicated to improving the quality of life of people with eczema and their carers.

Peanut Allergy UK

peanutallergyuk.co.uk

A support website for peanut allergy sufferers.

Talk Eczema

talkhealthpartnership.com/talkeczema/

A helpful eczema site including an A-Z of treatments, a newsletter, chat room and lots of information.

IN THE US

Celiac Disease Foundation

celiac.org

Celiac Disease Foundation provides a wide range of helpful information about living a gluten-free life in the US.

Go Dairy Free

godairyfree.org

A helpful support site for anyone on a dairy-free diet, with lots of recipes and product information.

Kids with Food Allergies

kidswithfoodallergies.org

This food allergy organization promotes the optimal health, nutrition, and wellbeing of children with food allergies by providing education and a support community for their families and caregivers.

OTHER LOCATIONS

Coeliac Ireland

coeliac.ie

Support and information for coeliacs in Ireland, from the country's national charity.

The Food Intolerance Group of Australia

foodintol.com

The website of this useful support group has a range of excellent information on food intolerances of all kinds.

References

Adlerberth I *et al*, "Gut microbiota and development of atopic eczema in 3 European birth cohorts", *Journal of Allergy and Clinical Immunology*. 2007; 120: 343–50.

Akobeng AK *et al*, "Effect of breast feeding on risk of celiac disease: a systematic review and meta-analysis of observational studies", *Archive of Disease in Childhood*. 2006; 91: 39–43.

Alduraywish SA *et al*, "Sensitization to milk, egg and peanut from birth to 18 years: A longitudinal study of a cohort at risk of allergic disease", *Pediatric Allergy and Immunology*. 2016 Feb; 27(1): 83–91.

Allen SJ *et al*, "Dietary supplementation with lactobacilli and bifidobacteria is well tolerated and not associated with adverse events during late pregnancy and early infancy". *Journal of Nutrition*. 2010 Mar; 140(3): 483–8.

Anagnostou K, Orange JS, "The Value of Food Allergy Prevention in Clinical Practice in Pediatrics: Targeting Early Life", *Children*. 2018; 5(2): 14.

Atkinson *et al*. "Food elimination based on IgG antibodies in irritable bowel syndrome: a randomised controlled trial", *Gut*. 2004; 53: 1459–64.

Bahna SL, Burkhardt JG, "The dilemma of allergy to food additives", *Allergy and Asthma Proceedings*. 2018 Jan; 39(1) 3–8.

Balmer JE, Blomhoff R, "Gene expression regulation by retinoic acid", *Journal of Lipid Research*. 2002 Nov; 43(11): 1773–1808.

Barachetti *et al*, "Weaning and complementary feeding in preterm infants: management, timing and health outcome", *La Pediatria Medica e Chirurgica*. 2017 Dec; 39(4): 181.

Birkenfeld S *et al*, "Celiac disease associated with psoriasis", *British Journal of Dermatology*. 2009; 161(6), 1331–4.

Brandtzaeg P, "Food allergy: separating the science from the mythology", *Nature Reviews: Gastroenterology and Hepatology*. 2010 Jul; 7(7): 380–400.

Brehm JM *et al*, "Childhood Asthma Management Program Research Group. Serum vitamin D levels and severe asthma exacerbations in the Childhood Asthma Management Program study". *J Allergy Clin Immunol.* 2010 Jul; 126(1): 52–8.

Brydon *et al*, "Peripheral inflammation is associated with altered substantia nigra activity and psychomotor slowing in humans", *Biological Psychiatry*. 2008 Jun; 63(11): 1022–9

Burk SA, Sampson HA, "Diagnostic approaches to the patient with suspected food allergies", *Journal of Pediatrics*. 1992 November; 121(5): S64–S71.

Burkitt DP, "Epidemiology of large bowel disease: The role of fibre", *The Proceedings of the Nutrition Society*. 1973 Dec; 32(3): 145–9.

Chawes BL *et al*, "Allergic sensitization at school age is a systemic low-grade inflammatory disorder", *Allergy*. 2017 Jul; 72(7): 1073–80.

Christian P, Stewart CP, "Maternal micronutrient deficiency, fetal development, and the risk of chronic disease", *J Nutr*. 2010 Mar; 140(3):437–45.

Clark AT *et al*, "Successful oral tolerance induction in severe peanut allergy", *Allergy*. 2009 Aug; 64(8): 1218–20.

Clausen M *et al*, "Fish oil in infancy protects against food allergy in Iceland–Results from a birth cohort study". *Allergy*. 2018 Jan 10. [Epub ahead of print]

Conrad ML *et al*, "Maternal TLR signaling is required for prenatal asthma protection by the nonpathogenic microbe *Acinetobacter lwoffii F78*", *Journal of Experimental Medicine*. 2009 Dec; 206(13): 2869.

Cummins AG, Thompson FM, "Postnatal changes in mucosal immune response: a physiological perspective of breast feeding and weaning", *Immunology and Cell Biology*. 1997 Oct; 75(5), 419–29.

Dahdah L *et al*, "How to predict and improve prognosis of food allergy". *Current Opinion in Allergy and Clinical Immunology*. 2018 Jun; 18(3): 228–33.

Dial EJ *et al*, "Oral phosphatidylcholine preserves gastrointestinal mucosal barrier during LPS-induced inflammation", *Shock*. 2008; 30(6): 729–33.

Dogan Y *et al*, "Prevalence of celiac disease among first-degree relatives of patients with celiac disease", *Journal of Pediatric Gastroenterology and Nutrition*. 2012 Aug; 55(2): 205–8.

Drago L *et al*, "Treatment of atopic dermatitis eczema with a high concentration of Lactobacillus salivarius LS01 associated with an innovative gelling complex: a pilot study on adults", *Journal of Clinical Gastroenterology*. 2014 Nov; 48(1): S47–51.

Drago L *et al*, "Effects of Lactobacillus salivarius LS01 (DSM 22775) treatment on adult atopic dermatitis: a randomized placebo-controlled study", *International Journal of Immunopathology and Pharmacology*. 2011 Oct; 24(4): 1037–48.

Dupont C *et al*, "Nutritional management of cow's milk allergy in children: An update", *Archives de Pediatrie*. 2018 Apr; 25(3): 236–243

Egger J *et al*, "Is migraine food allergy? A double-blind controlled trial of oligoantigenic diet treatment", *Lancet*. 1983 Oct; 15(2): 865–9.

Favre L *et al*, "Secretory IgA possesses intrinsic modulatory properties stimulating mucosal and systemic immune responses", *Journal of Immunology*. 2005 Sep; 175(5), 2793–2800.

De Filippo C *et al*, "Impact of diet in shaping gut microbiota revealed by a comparative study in children from Europe and rural Africa", *Proceedings of the National Academy of Sciences of the United States of America*. 2010 Aug; 107(33) 14691–6.

Finamore A *et al*, "Zinc may contribute to the host defense by maintaining the membrane barrier", *J Nutr*. 2008 Sep; 138(9):1664–70.

Fong AT *et al*, "Bullying and quality of life in children and adolescents with food allergy", *Journal of Paediatrics and Child Health*. 2017 Jul; 53(7): 630–5.

Forastiere F *et al*, "Consumption of fresh fruit rich in vitamin C and wheezing symptoms in children", *Thorax*. 2000 Apr; 55(4): 283–288.

Forsberg A *et al*, "Pre- and probiotics for allergy prevention: time to revisit recommendations?" *Clinical and Experimental Allergy*. 2016 Dec; 46(12): 1506–21.

Garcia-Larsen V *et al*, "Diet during pregnancy and infancy and risk of allergic or autoimmune disease: A systematic review and meta-analysis", *PLoS Medicine*. 2018 Feb; 15(2): e1002507.

Giannetti E, Staiano A, "Probiotics for Irritable Bowel Syndrome: Clinical Data in Children", *J Pediatr Gastroenterol Nutr*. 2016 Jul; 63(Suppl 1): S25–6.

Gil F *et al*, "Association between Caesarean Delivery and Isolated Doses of Formula Feeding in Cow Milk Allergy", *International Archives of Allergy and Immunology*. 2017; 173(3): 147–52.

Godfrey KM, Barker DJ, "Fetal nutrition and adult disease", *American Journal of Clinical Nutrition.* 2000 May; 71(5 Suppl): 1344S–52S.

Goldsmith AJ *et al*, "Formula and breast feeding in infant food allergy: A population-based study", *Journal of Paediatrics and Child Health.* 2016 Apr; 52(4): 377–84.

Greer FR *et al*, "Effects of early nutritional interventions on the development of atopic disease in infants and children: the role of maternal dietary restriction, breastfeeding, timing of introduction of complementary foods, and hydrolyzed formulas", *Pediatrics.* 2008 Jan; 121(1): 183–91.

Guo H *et al*, "Correlation between serum vitamin D status and immunological changes in children affected by gastrointestinal food allergy", *Allergologia et Immunopathologia.* 2018 Jan; 46(1): 39–44.

Hallert C *et al*, "Evidence of poor vitamin status in celiac patients on a gluten-free diet for 10 years", *Alimentary Pharmacology and Therapeutics.* 2002 Jul; 16(1): 1333–9.

Hamer HM *et al*, "Review article: the role of butyrate on colonic function", *Aliment Pharmacol Ther.* 2008 Jan; 27(2): 104–19.

Hardman G, Hart G, "Dietary advice based on food-specific IgG results", *Nutrition & Food Science.* 2007; 37(1): 16–23.

Helms S, "Celiac disease and gluten associated diseases", *Alternative Medicine Review.* 2005 Sep; 10(3): 172–92.

Henriksson C *et al*, "What effect does breastfeeding have on coeliac disease? A systematic review update", *Evidence-Based Medicine.* 2013 Jun; 18(3): 98–103.

Hilty M *et al*, "Disordered microbial communities in asthmatic airways", *PLoS One.* 2010 Jan; 5(1):e8578.

Holt PG, Strickland DH, "Soothing signals: transplacental transmission of resistance to asthma and allergy", *J Exp Med.* 2009 Dec; 206(13): 2861–4.

Hoppu U *et al*, "Maternal diet rich in saturated fat during breastfeeding is associated with atopic sensitization of the infant", *European Journal of Clinical Nutrition.* 2000 Jan; 54(9): 702–5.

Høst A. "Cow's milk protein allergy and intolerance in infancy. Some clinical, epidemiological and immunological aspects", *Pediatr Allergy Immunol.* 1994; 5(5 Suppl): 1–36.

Høst A *et al*, "Dietary prevention of allergic diseases in infants and small children", *Pediatr Allergy Immunol.* 2008 Feb; 19(1): 1–4.

Huurre A *et al*, "Impact of maternal atopy and probiotic supplementation during pregnancy on infant sensitization: a double-blind placebo-controlled study", *Clinical and Experimental Allergy.* 2008 Aug; 38(8): 1342–8.

Ierodiakonou D *et al*, "Timing of Allergenic Food Introduction to the Infant Diet and Risk of Allergic or Autoimmune Disease: A Systematic Review and Meta-analysis", *JAMA.* 2016 Sep; 316(11): 1181–92.

Iikura *et al*, "How to prevent allergic disease. I. Study of specific IgE, IgG, and IgG4 antibodies in serum of pregnant mothers, cord blood, and infants", *International Archives of Allergy and Applied Immunology.* 1989; 88(1-2): 250–2.

Imler JL, Hoffmann JA, "Toll receptors in innate immunity", *Trends in Cell Biology.* 2001 Jul; 11(7), 304–11.

Incorvaia C *et al*, "Allergic rhinitis", *Journal of Biological Regulators and Homeostatic Agents.* 2018 Jan; 32(1 Suppl. 1): 61–6.

Inuoe R *et al*, "A preliminary study of gut dysbiosis in children with food allergy", *Bioscience, Biotechnology, Biochemistry.* 2017 Dec; 81(12): 2396–99.

Jalonen T, "Identical permeability changes in children with different clinical manifestations of cow's milk allergy", *J Allergy Clin Immunol.* 1991 Nov; 88(5): 737–42.

Janzi M *et al.* "Selective IgA deficiency in early life: association to infections and allergic diseases during childhood", *Clinical Immunology.* 2009 Oct; 133(1): 78–85.

Jiménez E *et al*, "Isolation of commensal bacteria from umbilical cord blood of healthy neonates born by cesarean section", *Current Microbiology.* 2005 Oct; 51(4): 270–4.

Johnson CC *et al*, "Antibiotic exposure in early infancy and risk for childhood atopy", *J Allergy Clin Immunol.* 2005 Jun; 115(6): 1218–24.

Kagalwalla AF *et al*, "Efficacy of a 4-Food Elimination Diet for Children With Eosinophilic Esophagitis", *Clinical Gastroenterololgy and Hepatology.* 2017 Nov; 15(11): 1698–1707.

Kankaanpää P *et al*, "Dietary fatty acids and allergy", *Annals of Medicine.* 1999 Aug; 31(4): 282–7.

Karabacak E *et al*, "Erythrocyte zinc level in patients with atopic dermatitis and its relation to SCORAD index", *Postepy dermatologii i alergologii*. 2016 Oct; 33(5): 349–52.

von Kobyletzki LB *et al*, "Association between childhood allergic diseases, educational attainment and occupational status in later life: systematic review protocol", *BMJ Open*. 2017 Oct; 7.

Kong J *et al*, "Novel role of the vitamin D receptor in maintaining the integrity of the intestinal mucosal barrier", *American Journal of Physiology – Gastrointestinal and Liver Physiology*. 2008 Jan; 294(1): G208–16

König J *et al*, "Human Intestinal Barrier Function in Health and Disease", *Clinical and Translational Gastroenterology*. 2016 Oct; 7(10): e196.

Krzych-Fałta E *et al*, "Probiotics: Myths or facts about their role in allergy prevention", *Advances in Clinical and Experimental Medicine*. 2018 Jan; 27(1): 119–24.

Lack G, "Epidemiologic risks for food allergy", *J Allergy Clin Immunol*. 2008 Jun; 121(6): 1331–6.

Laffont S, Powrie F, "Immunology: Dendritic-cell genealogy", *Nature*. 2009 Dec; 462: 732–3.

Larson K *et al*, "Introducing Allergenic Food into Infants' Diets: Systematic Review", *MCN. The American Journal of Maternal Child Nursing*. 2017 Mar/Apr; 42(2): 72–80.

Latvala S *et al*, "Potentially probiotic bacteria induce efficient maturation but differential cytokine production in human monocyte-derived dendritic cells", *World Journal of Gastroenterology*. 2008 Sep; 14(36): 5570–83.

Ley RE *et al*, "Microbial ecology: Human gut microbes associated with obesity", *Nature* 444: 1022–1023.

Litonjua A, Weiss S, "Is vitamin D deficiency to blame for the asthma epidemic?" *J Allergy Clin Immunol*. 2007 Nov; 120(5): 1031–5.

Liu AH, Leung DY, "Renaissance of the hygiene hypothesis", *J Allergy Clin Immunol*. 2006 May; 117(5): 1063–6.

Lucarelli S *et al*, "Specific IgG and IgA Antibodies and Related Subclasses in the Diagnosis of Gastrointestinal Disorders or Atopic Dermatitis Due to Cow's Milk and Egg",

International Journal of Immunopathology and Pharmacology. 1998 May; 11(2): 77–85.

Ly NP *et al*, "Gut microbiota, probiotics, and vitamin D: Interrelated exposures influencing allergy, asthma, and obesity?" *J Allergy Clin Immunol.* 2011 March; 127(5): 1087–94.

Magnusson J *et al*, "Fish and polyunsaturated fat intake and development of allergic and nonallergic rhinitis", *J Allergy Clin Immunol.* 2015 Jul; 136(5): 1247–53

Majamaa H *et al*, "Probiotics: a novel approach in the management of food allergy", *J Allergy Clin Immunol.* 1997 Feb; 99(2): 179–85.

Malterre T, "Digestive and Nutritional Considerations in Celiac Disease: Could Supplementation Help?" *Alternative Medicine Review.* 2009 Sep; 14(3): 247–57.

Martin R *et al*, "The commensal microflora of human milk: new perspectives for food bacteriotherapy and probiotics", *Trends in Food Science and Technology.* 2003 Mar; 15(3): 121–7.

Maslowski K, Mackay C, "Diet, gut microbiota and immune responses", *Nature Immunology.* 2011 Jan; 12(1): 5–9.

Mavroudi A *et al*, "Assessment of IgE-mediated food allergies in children with atopic dermatitis", *Allergologia et Immunopathologia.* 2017 Jan/Feb; 45(1): 77–81.

Mayer L, "Mucosal immunity", *Pediatrics.* 2003 Jun; 111(6 Pt 3): 1595–600.

McGowan KE *et al*, "The Changing Face of Childhood Celiac Disease in North America: Impact of Serological Testing", *Pediatrics.* 2009 Dec; 124(6): 1572–8.

Mermiri DT *et al*, "Review suggests that the immunoregulatory and anti-inflammatory properties of allergenic foods can provoke oral tolerance if introduced early to infants' diets", *Acta Paediatrica.* 2017 May; 106(5): 721–6.

Meyer U *et al*, "Immunological stress at the maternal-foetal interface: a link between neurodevelopment and adult psychopathology", *Brain Behavior and Immunity.* 2006 Jul; 20(4): 378–88.

Miles EA, Calder PC, "Can Early Omega-3 Fatty Acid Exposure Reduce Risk of Childhood Allergic Disease?" *Nutrients.* 2017 Jul; 9(7): 784.

Mira A *et al*, "The Neolithic revolution of bacterial genomes", *Trends in Microbiology.* 2006 May; 14(5):200–6.

Miraglia Del Giudice M *et al*, "Probiotics and Allergic Respiratory Diseases", *J Biol Regul Homeost Agents.* 2015 Apr–Jun; 29(2 Suppl 1): 80–3.

Mitchell N *et al*, "Randomised controlled trial of food elimination diet based on IgG antibodies for the prevention of migraine like headaches", *Nutrition*. 2011 Aug; 10: 85.

Mondoulet L *et al*, "Specific epicutaneous immunotherapy prevents sensitization to new allergens in a murine model", *J Allergy Clin Immunol*. 2015 Jun; 135(6): 1546–57.

Mösges R *et al*, "Short-course of grass allergen peptides immunotherapy over three weeks reduces seasonal symptoms in allergic rhinoconjunctivitis with/without Asthma: A randomized, multicenter, double-blind, placebo-controlled trial", *Allergy*. 2018 Mar 7. [Epub ahead of print]

Mucida D *et al*, "From the diet to the nucleus: vitamin A and TGF-beta join efforts at the mucosal interface of the intestine", *Seminars in Immunology*. 2009 Feb; 21(1):14–21.

Muluk NB, Cingi C, "Oral allergy syndrome", *American Journal of Rhinology and Allergy*. 2018 Jan; 32(1): 27–30.

Nadal I *et al*, "Imbalance in the composition of the duodenal microbiota of children with celiac disease", *Journal of Medical Microbiology*. 2007 Mar; 56(12): 1669–74.

Ng N *et al*, "House dust extracts have both TH2 adjuvant and tolerogenic activities", *J Allergy Clin Immunol*. 2006 May; 117(5): 1074–81.

Nicolaou N *et al*, "Reintroduction of cow's milk in milk-allergic children", *Endocrine, Metabolic and Immune Disorders Drug Targets*. 2014 Mar; 14(1): 54–62.

Niers L *et al*, "The effects of selected probiotic strains on the development of eczema (the PandA study)", *Allergy*. 2009 Sep; 64(9): 1349–58.

Niers L *et al*, "Selection of probiotic bacteria for prevention of allergic diseases: immunomodulation of neonatal dendritic cells", *Clinical and Experimental Immunology*. 2007 Aug; 149(2): 344–52.

Novembre E *et al*, "Milk allergy/intolerance and atopic dermatitis in infancy and childhood", *Allergy*. 2001; 56 (Suppl 67): 105–8.

Noverr M, Huffnagle G, "Does the microbiota regulate immune responses outside the gut?" *Trends Microbiol*. 2004 Dec; 12(12): 562–8.

Nurmatov U *et al*, "Nutrients and foods for the primary prevention of asthma and allergy: Systematic review and meta-analysis", *J Allergy Clin Immunol*. 2011 Mar; 127(3): 724–33.

Oranje AP *et al*, "Natural course of cow's milk allergy in childhood atopic eczema/dermatitis syndrome", *Annals of Allergy, Asthma and Immunology*. 2002 Dec; 89(6 Suppl 1): 52–5.

Oriel RC *et al*,"How to manage food allergy in nursery or school", *Curr Opin Allergy Clin Immunol*. 2018 Jun; 18(3): 258–64. [ahead of Print: Mar 2018]

Palmer DJ, Makrides M, "Diet of lactating women and allergic reactions in their infants", *Current Opinion in Clinical Nutrition and Metabolic Care*. 2006 May; 9(3), 284–8.

van Parijs L, Abbas AK, "Homeostasis and self-tolerance in the immune system: turning lymphocytes off", *Science*. 1998 Apr; 280(5361): 243–8.

Patel N *et al*, "The emotional, social, and financial burden of food allergies on children and their families", *Allergy and Asthma Proceedings*. 2017 Mar; 38(2): 88–91.

I Pavić *et al*, "Growth of Children with Food Allergy", *Hormone Research in Paediatrics*. 2017; 88(1): 91–100.

Penders J *et al*, "The role of the intestinal microbiota in the development of atopic disorders", *Allergy*. 2007 Nov; 62(11): 1223–36.

Perezabad L *et al*, "The establishment of cow's milk protein allergy in infants is related with a deficit of regulatory T cells (Treg) and vitamin D", *Pediatric Research*. 2017 May; 81(5): 722–30.

Pessi T *et al*, "Interleukin-10 generation in atopic children following oral Lactobacillus rhamnosus GG", *Clin Exp Allergy*. 2000 Dec; 30(12): 1804–8.

Pinto-Sánchez MI *et al*, "Gluten Introduction to Infant Feeding and Risk of Celiac Disease: Systematic Review and Meta-Analysis", *J Pediatr.* 2016 Jan; 168: 132–43.

Poole A *et al*, "Cellular and molecular mechanisms of vitamin D in food allergy", *Journal of Cellular and Molecular Medicine*. 2018 Mar 25. [Epub ahead of print]

Prescott SL *et al*, "Supplementation with Lactobacillus rhamnosus or Bifidobacterium lactis probiotics in pregnancy increases cord blood interferon-gamma and breast milk transforming growth factor-beta and immunoglobin A detection", *Clin Exp Allergy*. 2009 May; 39(5): 771.

Ramagopalan SV *et al*, "A ChIP-seq defined genome-wide map of vitamin D receptor binding: associations with disease and evolution", *Genome Research*. 2010 Oct; 20(10): 1352–60.

Rees T *et al*, "A Prospective Audit of Food Intolerance Among Migraine Patients in Primary Care Clinical Practice", *Headache Care*. 2005; 2(1): 11–14.

Resnick C, "Nutritional Protocol for the Treatment of Intestinal Permeability Defects and Related Conditions", *Natural Medicine Journal*. 2010 March; 2(3).

Rook GA, Brunet LR, "Microbes, immunoregulation, and the gut", *Gut*. 2005 Mar; 54(3): 317–20.

Rook GA, "Review series on helminths, immune modulation and the hygiene hypothesis: The broader implications of the hygiene hypothesis Immunology", 2009 Jan; 126 (1), 3–11.

Rosenfeldt V *et al*, "Effect of probiotics on gastrointestinal symptoms and small intestinal permeability in children with atopic dermatitis", *J Pediatr*. 2004 Nov; 145(5): 612–16.

Rubio-Tapia A *et al*, "Increased prevalence and mortality in undiagnosed celiac disease", *Gastroenterology*. 2009 Jul; 137(1): 88–93.

Ruemmele FM *et al*, "Clinical evidence for immunomodulatory effects of probiotic bacteria", *J Pediatr Gastroenterol Nutr*. 2009 Feb; 48(2): 126–41.

Sapone A *et al*, "Spectrum of gluten-related disorders: consensus on new nomenclature and classification", *BMC Medicine*. 2012 Feb; 10(1):13.

Schouten B *et al*, "Cow milk allergy symptoms are reduced in mice fed dietary synbiotics during oral sensitization with whey", *J Nutr*. 2009 Jul; 139(7): 1398–403.

Shoda T *et al*, "Yogurt consumption in infancy is inversely associated with atopic dermatitis and food sensitization at 5 years of age: A hospital-based birth cohort study", *Journal of Dermatological Science*. 2017 May; 86(2), 90–6.

Smits HH *et al*, "Selective probiotic bacteria induce IL-10-producing regulatory T cells in vitro by modulating dendritic cell function through dendritic cell-specific intercellular adhesion molecule 3-grabbing nonintegrin", *J Allergy Clin Immunol*. 2005 Jun; 115(6): 1260–7.

Sommer A, "Vitamin A deficiency and clinical disease: An historical overview", *J Nutr*. 2008 Oct; 138(10): 1835–39.

Strachan DP, "Hay fever, hygiene, and household size", *British Medical Journal* 1989 Nov; 299 (6710): 1259–60.

Strober W, "Vitamin A rewrites the ABCs of oral tolerance", *Mucosal Immunology*. 2008 Mar; 1(2): 92–5.

Suzuki K, Fagarasan S, "Diverse regulatory pathways for IgA synthesis in the gut", *Mucosal Immunology*. 2009 Nov; 2(6): 468–71.

Szajewska H *et al*, "Gluten Introduction and the Risk of Coeliac Disease: A Position Paper by the European Society for Pediatric Gastroenterology, Hepatology, and Nutrition", *J Pediatr Gastroenterol Nutr*. 2016 Mar; 62(3): 507–13.

Szajewska H *et al*, "Systematic review: early infant feeding and the prevention of coeliac disease", *Aliment Pharmacol Ther*. 2012 Oct; 36(7): 607–18.

Täljemark J *et al*, "The coexistence of psychiatric and gastrointestinal problems in children with restrictive eating in a nationwide Swedish twin study", *Journal of Eating Disorders*. 2017 Aug; 5: 25.

Tanaka M *et al*, "Signatures in the gut microbiota of Japanese infants who developed food allergies in early childhood", *FEMS Microbiology Ecology*. 2017 Aug; 93(8).

Taniuchi S *et al*, "Dual Factors May Be Necessary for Development of Atopic March in Early Infancy", *Journal of Nippon Medical School*. 2018; 85: 2–10.

Tariq SM *et al*, "The prevalence of and risk factors for atopy in early childhood: a whole population birth cohort study", *J Allergy Clin Immunol*. 1998 May; 101(5): 587–93.

Du Toit, G *et al*, "Early consumption of peanuts in infancy is associated with a low prevalence of peanut allergy", *J. Allergy Clin. Immunol*. 2008 Nov; 122(5): 984–91.

Du Toit G *et al*, "Randomized trial of peanut consumption in infants at risk for peanut allergy", *New England Journal of Medicine*. 2015 Feb; 372(9): 803–13.

Toomer OT *et al*, "Maternal and postnatal dietary probiotic supplementation enhances splenic regulatory T helper cell population and reduces ovalbumin allergen-induced hypersensitivity responses in mice", *Immunobiology*. 2014 May; 219(5): 367–76.

Turati F *et al*, "Early weaning is beneficial to prevent atopic dermatitis occurrence in young children", *Allergy*. 2016 Jun; 71(6): 878–88.

Turke PW, "Childhood food allergies An evolutionary mismatch hypothesis", *Evolultion, Medicine and Public Health*. 2017 Oct; 1: 154–160.

Untersmayr E *et al*, "Antacid medication inhibits digestion of dietary proteins and causes food allergy: a fish allergy model in BALB/c mice", *J. Allergy Clin. Immunol.* 2003 Sep; 112(3): 616–23.

Venkataraman D *et al*, "Prevalence and longitudinal trends of food allergy during childhood and adolescence: Results of the Isle of Wight Birth Cohort study", *Clin Exp Allergy*. 2018 Apr; 48(4): 394–402.

Venter C *et al*, "Impact of elimination diets on nutrition and growth in children with multiple food allergies", *Curr Opin Allergy Clin Immunol.* 2017 Jun; 17(3): 220–6.

Verhasselt V, "Oral tolerance in neonates: from basics to potential prevention of allergic disease", *Mucosal Immunology*. 2010 Jul; 3(4), 326–33.

Vojdani A, Tarash I, "Cross-Reaction between Gliadin and Different Food and Tissue Antigens", *Food and Nutrition Sciences*. 2013 Jan; 4(1): 20–32.

Walker MT *et al*, "Mechanism for initiation of food allergy: Dependence on skin barrier mutations and environmental allergen costimulation", *J Allergy Clin Immunol.* 2018 Feb 15. [Ebook ahead of print]

Wegienka G *et al*, "Lifetime dog and cat exposure and dog- and cat-specific sensitization at age 18 years", *Clin Exp Allergy*. 2011 Jul; 41(7): 979–86.

Wichers H, "Immunomodulation by food: promising concept for mitigating allergic disease?" *Analalytical and Bioanalytical Chemistry*. 2009 Sep; 395(1): 37–45.

Willemsen LE *et al*, "Polyunsaturated fatty acids support epithelial barrier integrity and reduce IL-4 mediated permeability in vitro", *European Journal of Nutrition*. 2008 Jun; 47(4): 183–191.

Zioudrou C *et al*, "Opioid peptides derived from food proteins: The exorphins." *Journal of Biological Chemistry*. 1979 Apr; 254(7): 2446–9.

Index

Acknowledgments

A special thank you to my husband who provides ongoing support and encouragement for all the work I do. I would particularly like to thank the team at Watkins: Kate Fox, Dan Hurst, Judy Barratt, Georgina Hewitt, Lucia Garavaglia and Vikki Scott for the thought and sheer hard work they have put into producing this book.

About the Author

CHRISTINE BAILEY is an award-winning nutritionist, IFM functional nutrition practitioner, food consultant, chef and cookery teacher. She runs two clinics, including one on Harley Street, provides nutritional support to corporates, health-food companies and local authorities, hosts cookery days and lectures on nutrition. A member of the Guild of Health Writers, Christine also writes for numerous health and food magazines and her books include *The Supercharged Green Juice & Smoothie Diet*, *Supercharged Juice & Smoothie Recipes*, *The Raw Food Diet* and *The Gut Health Diet Plan.*

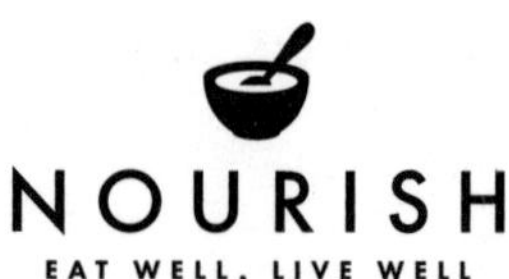
NOURISH
EAT WELL, LIVE WELL